T0284262

TOMORROW'S
WEIGH

THE NO-DIET WAY
TO LOSE WEIGHT

TOMORROW'S WEIGH

The No-Diet Way to Lose Weight

© 2024,

Richard R. Terry, DO, MBA

Helen E. Battisti, PHD, RDN

Francis L. Battisti, PHD, MSW

Print ISBN: 979-8-35095-613-9

eBook ISBN: 979-8-35095-614-6

CONTENTS

INTRODUCTION

What This Book Is NOT

This is not a book about dieting. It's about starvation.

STARVATION IS A STRANGE PHENOMENON TO FEATURE so prominently in the 21st century in the wealthiest nation on the planet, but there is no other word for the culture of weight consciousness and weight loss that pervades every corner of our daily lives.

Starvation is the silent culprit. It's the skeletal models defining our concepts of beauty in magazines, movies, and media. It's the fat-free, carb-free, keto, zero-calorie choices on the supermarket shelves. It's the rise in eating disorders among pre-pubescent children and the increase of diabetes and pre-diabetes in our adolescents.

Self-Help Doesn't Help

There are hundreds of diet books on the self-help shelves of every brick-and-mortar bookstore or bookselling website. The American weight-loss industry grosses $71 billion in revenue every year. Forty-nine percent of adults report being on a diet the previous year. And all the while, the percentage of adults who are overweight or obese continues to increase (currently at 73%). Even our children are not immune from this trend: 41% of them fall into one of these two categories as well. These statistics cost a fortune in obesity-related health care and broken, despairing lives. And it's getting worse, not better.

This is not a coincidence. There is no logical way that using words like "sinful" to talk about eating certain foods, idolizing ultra-thin images, and applauding fat-to-thin celebrity stories the way our grandparents glorified rags-to-riches tales could not be related to the fact that we are growing increasingly obese. We are getting fatter, not despite the fact that we are encouraged to eat less, but *because* of it.

Americans are starving themselves, dieting more, yet still weighing more. We have indeed become a "starvation nation."

What This Book Is

So, if this is not a self-help diet book, what is it? It's a concise, readable look at the shocking news that our very attitudes, social mores, popular culture, and even misdirected aspects of our increasing attention to health are sabotaging our hopes and dreams of living fit, energetic lifestyles. Whole segments of our population have forced themselves into at-risk eating behaviors, setting up situations where even dieters with the best-intentions are doomed to failure.

Take-Home Points

- Dieting makes you fat.
- You can lose weight by eating.
- There are no such things as "bad" or "good" foods.

Reflection Questions

1. If you've ever used a restrictive diet, did it have long-term results?

2. Who are you making lifestyle changes for, and why?

3. What's the number-one lifestyle choice you want to work on—increasing physical activity? Making healthier food choices? Getting more sleep? Something else?

CHAPTER 1

YOUR PROBLEM...
AND HOW TO SOLVE IT

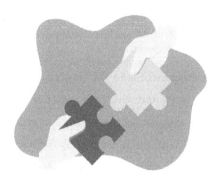

LET'S GET ONE THING STRAIGHT: IN YOUR HEART OF hearts, you must want to lose weight for good. You must want to be happier. You must want to live longer and be healthier.

You must *want* to enjoy your meals and snacks MORE and not less. You must *want* the sense of confidence, pride and well-being that comes with regular physical activity. You must admit the possibility that fad dieting is not going to work—ever—and learn the rock-solid reasons why that is so.

The first step in any self-improvement program is to accept yourself and your body as it really is without any self-hating hang-ups about how you appear to yourself or others, or how much you weigh. These are things—body type, bone structure, genes—that you cannot change. But tell yourself you're going to work on the things that you can change: weight, personal health condition, eating habits, physical activity, and, finally and most importantly, the lifestyle that allows you to exist in the first place.

The second requirement is that you stop all fad dieting now— right now. Stop even thinking about dieting. Prepare to reject all future dieting magic bullets, the "no this" and "no that" fad diets of any kind. There are no new discoveries on how to lose weight with or without dieting.

The third requirement is to start eating. Start eating well. Not tomorrow, not next week, but with your very next meal. Never starve yourself again. And you won't. Because this program will help you decide *how* to eat, *how much* to eat, and *when* to eat, but not *what* to eat. You will make that choice. We will offer you alternatives to those suggestions. We will help you find your own alternatives, but we will never permit you to starve yourself again—and, when you see and feel the results to be gained by following the Tomorrow's Weigh® nutritional and activity program, you will feel wonderful—about yourself, about your body, about your food, your sleep, your confident personality, and your physical activity program. What's more, you'll be preparing, eating and enjoying all the food you need or want for the rest of your healthy life!

Look at what is on the menu for your very next meal. Is it chock full of sugar? Is it something you know you can't stop eating, even though you are satisfied? Is it all highly processed? Is it a pickup from a fast food? If possible, discard those destructive choices on today's menu. If not, enjoy your next meal—whatever it consists of right now—because that's the way you will be enjoying your meals after you get with the program. However, if it's processed, sugary, addictive, or a fast food "quickie," let it be the last. Because you're going to change all that.

The fourth requirement is preparing to accept a regular exercise regimen. It might begin with just stretching, breathing, walking, swimming, or basic cardio. Whatever it is, you should plan on having your primary care provider's approval. Soon you will start the training necessary to discard excess fat and build lean muscle. You'll notice an improvement in heart rate and breathing fairly quickly and, most of all, you'll start to really enjoy it.

The fifth requirement is to get ready to limit your screen time (TV and devices), jumping in the car for even short distances, and totally relying on household gadgets for every single chore such as vacuuming, washing dishes, or mowing the lawn.

If you have some physical limitations, you know how much you can do. But whatever your circumstances are, you can start to stretch, breathe right, pay attention to what you eat, enjoy it more, and assume a style of living that leads to a longer and more fulfilling life. That's what this program is about—not only your Tomorrow's Weigh®, but also your lifestyle today and tomorrow.

Why Diets Don't Work

When physiologist Dr. Ancel Keys (he's the K in Army "K rations") and his colleagues at the University of Minnesota began a study in the fall of 1944, it wasn't dieting they were concerned with: They were compiling data for the U.S. government to assist with famine relief in Europe and Asia.

Keys placed 32 conscientious objectors to the ongoing war—all healthy young men used to eating hearty meals—on a voluntary "semi-starvation" diet of 1,570 calories a day. (That's less than half of what they were used to eating, but much higher than the 1,000–1,200 calorie fad diets touted today in most women's magazines.)

When the starvation program ended at the six-month mark, participants' metabolism slowed, with an average drop of about 40% at the end of the six months. Additionally, they felt cold, weak, tired, and became obsessed with food, even collecting recipes, planning menus and studying cookbooks! Further, they became depressed, anxious, irritable, and anti-social toward others in the group. Within three months they were eating normally again. However, they gained back more than half the weight they'd lost, and gained fat tissue instead of hard muscle. "Soft roundness" was their new body type. Yes, they had lost pounds, but it came back on as increased fat.

The men also became binge eaters: They could not seem to satisfy themselves and ate to the point of being stuffed. They not only gained their lost pounds back, but continued to overeat and gained additional weight well after the study ended. The title of Dr. Keys' 1950 book on the study? *The Biology of Human Starvation.*

As participants continued to eat again, some of their symptoms went away. But long-term effects lingered, including binge eating, and made it difficult to manage their weight although they had never had weight concerns prior to the study.

Take-Home Point

• Diets lead to short-term weight loss. To sustain weight loss, you must undergo a lifestyle change.

Reflection Questions

1. How do you feel about your body? Do you know what outside influences created your relationship with your appearance?

2. What is a potential barrier—mental, time, monetary or otherwise—that might prevent you from making lifestyle changes?

3. What is an easy first step for you to make? Parking at the back of the lot to add extra steps? Adding in a walk at lunchtime? Something else?

CHAPTER 2

WHY WE DON'T RECOMMEND FAD DIETS OR ANY OTHER DIET PLANS

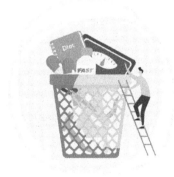

D **IETS ARE DANGEROUS. IN FACT, SOME DIETS CAN BE** killers.

Any diet plan other than a balanced, wholesome one either adds something your body doesn't need or, more often, deprives it of something it does need. Food marketers, authors, columnists, and even doctors shout about "no fat," "low fat," "low carb," "high protein," and "high fat" diets. However, take away those fats, carbohydrates, and proteins needed to nourish your body, and these starvation diets are life-threatening. They are life-threatening because the body sustains irreparable damage from severe malnutrition, eventually dies of hunger, or, after the diet becomes intolerable and regular eating resumes, causes compulsive overeating. As a result, the body regains the lost pounds, plus more. Worse, the body usually stores both the restored and the new pounds almost entirely as fat, not as the lean muscle lost in the diet phase.

This is due to glucose, better known as blood sugar. Certain parts of the body use only glucose for energy. When the body breaks down stored body fat, sufficient glucose isn't released and the body must get it from somewhere—so it breaks down lean muscle. The longer the dieting continues—especially if there aren't any muscle-building activities—the body slowly loses lean muscle.

Starvation diets take away what you need to renew your tissues, bones, muscles, skin and blood. They take away the energy you need to get through the day. Our bodies are designed to renew themselves, unless catastrophic illness, deprivation, or we ourselves interfere with that renewal.

Proteins, carbohydrates, and fats are the essentials that every individual needs to stay healthy and grow their tissues, bones, muscles, skin and blood. Meanwhile, huge food conglomerates with savvy marketing experts are having a heyday. They know a good thing when they see it on a sales chart. How about soft drinks? They are colored carbonated water, some labeled "sugar-free," meaning they have no energy benefits but chemical additives instead. The whole spectrum of diet products over the past 30 years has doubled, tripled and now quadrupled in sales. Book publishers can't put out more diet books fast enough. Television hosts, celebrities, and bloggers assault us with more guests touting magic weight-loss formulas and books. Commercials sell diet drugs, shakes, nutrition bars, drinks and "before and after" testimonials.

Frankly, if diets work, why is obesity on the rise? Why are we beginning to see an epidemic of Type II diabetes in children, teens, and adults? Simply, the widespread phenomenon of fad diets and the repeated myth of their benefits are pervasive in our culture. Many, if not most, diets are a form of starvation. Whenever your body loses something, nature makes up for it in some way or the living organism will die. In the case of fad dieting, the makeup happens through rebound overeating and weight gain.

The flab problem goes way beyond shame, guilt, and exhaustion. It causes people to make poor decisions, such as choosing a diet that utterly cuts out the needed balanced supply of proteins, carbohydrates, and fats. An example is skipping meals, rather than eating wholesomely three to five times a day. Another is lolling around, flopping down in front of the TV or device screen for hours, without any exercise day after day, or not even walking as far as the corner mailbox. People think they're solving their weight problems by cutting calories through the use of pills and diets. Every hour, every day, incorrect decisions about how to lose weight make people chronically tired and make them candidates for lifelong disease—and it's all because their bodies are starving.

You need a certain amount of energy just to live, think, eat, sleep, and breathe. The body is not like a furnace or stove which, when the fire goes out, just goes cold. Nature wants the body to live and survive whatever the circumstances. That's the whole purpose of life, and why we can survive deadly germs, why we heal, and even why we reproduce. So when the fuel isn't there, the body instinctively goes looking inside itself for the energy to survive.

First, it seeks out the vital blood sugar produced in the liver, because blood sugar fuels the most important organs in your body and your brain and serves the central nervous system. The survival of the brain and nervous system are the first priority. They are huge energy consumers, so they use up the liver as a first source.

Then the brain has to go looking elsewhere for more blood sugar. Where does it go? Not to the fat cells. They're good for energy for the rest of the body, but not for the blood sugar to use as "brain food." So, when the brain food isn't readily available from starches, dairy and fruit in your diet, and there's none remaining in the liver, then the brain goes looking for the tools it needs to make more blood sugar. Those tools are called amino acids, and it finds them by breaking down the proteins in lean muscle tissue.

Before you know it, the body is in a state of what doctors call ketosis (see box). This is precisely what happens to people in a famine, whether caused by natural or imposed consequences such as drought, poverty, or conflict. It seems horribly absurd, but that's exactly what some diet plans sell because clients register their starvation as weight loss when stepping on the scale.

Ketosis is an unnatural bodily state. When the body is deprived of carbohydrates, it looks to other sources such as stored fats or triglycerides. These are broken down in the blood in the form of ketones, which tend to mask appetite. Even though the brain demands glucose, ketosis results. This may cause symptoms such as headaches, light-headedness, and mental fatigue. Eventually, if you remain on such a diet, it will deplete fat stores and break down protein from your muscles to maintain energy. The onset of ketosis is a semi-starvation state.

Take-Home Point

- Any diets that induce ketosis are unhealthy.

Reflection Questions

1. If you've ever used a diet that induced ketosis, how did it make you feel?

2. What's your overall goal—to feel better? Live longer? Will your current lifestyle help you achieve this goal? What changes do you need to make?

3. Take a day and tally all the weight-loss messages you see, online, on billboards, in print, on television. How do encounters with these messages make you feel?

CHAPTER 3

YOUR WEIGHT AND HEALTH

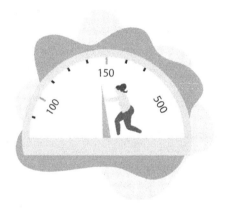

NEARLY TWO-THIRDS OF THE US POPULATION IS either overweight or obese. Every chronic medical condition from high blood pressure to gout can be linked to weight. World-wide, some four millions deaths per year are directly attributable to obesity.

Obesity decreases lifespan by almost four years and has replaced smoking as the number one globally-preventable disease. The data suggest obesity in childhood or adolescence is highly predictive of obesity in adulthood.

It's obvious that excess weight makes your heart work harder, which increases the chances of congestive heart failure, heart attack, or stroke. Chronic diseases like high blood pressure and diabetes both directly correlate with weight. In fact, 80% of patients with type 2 diabetes are overweight and could resolve their symptoms with weight loss. Sleep apnea—repeatedly stopping and starting breathing, which causes awakening and prevents fully restful sleep—is almost entirely due to obesity and, untreated, is a leading cause of early death. Abdominal fat (also known as visceral obesity, or fat around your organs like the heart, liver, and intestines) is major cause of the following conditions:

- Asthma

- Blood clots

- Dementia

- Gastroesophageal reflux disease (acid reflux)

- Heart problems (heart failure, heart attack, atrial fibrillation)

- Infertility (male and female)

- Intestinal cancer (cancer of the bowel, pancreas)

- Kidney disease (kidney failure or kidney stones)

- Liver disease (fatty liver disease and liver cancer)

- Lung disease

- Uterine cancer

Virtually every organ system in the body is affected by weight. Weight even affects the ability to fight infection: Being overweight impairs the immune system and makes the body more susceptible to bacterial and viral infections like influenza. The COVID pandemic demonstrated beyond a doubt that obesity is a substantial risk factor for major respiratory complications and death.

Excess weight also stresses the musculoskeletal system and can lead to osteoarthritis and chronic back pain. Insurance claims show that overweight or obese patients have twice than the absenteeism from work and almost twice the rate of disability claims. More subtle and less quantifiable are the effects of weight on the psyche. It's well-documented that obese patients have a higher risk of depression, anxiety, and other psychological diseases. Obesity carries a significant social stigma that affects economic potential and social status.

As we age, weight directly correlates to activity levels. The heavier you are, the less you move. The less you move, the more you gain. It's a vicious cycle and a literal death spiral.

Take-Home Point

- Most chronic medical conditions are due to excess weight and are curable with weight loss.

Reflection Questions

1. What are your thoughts about the global overweight and obesity reports?

2. Do you think your weight is limiting you in any way?

3. If so, what are you looking forward to as a result of your weight loss?

CHAPTER 4

FASTING OFF THE POUNDS:
FACT OR FICTION?

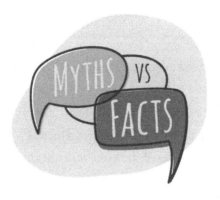

FASTING IS ALL THE RAGE NOW, BILLED AS A QUICK way to lose weight. The claim is that all you must do to lose a few pounds is a "simple" change in when you eat. Well, not so fast.

Many studies do support fasting as a weight-loss strategy. There are several popular fasting protocols ranging from an every other day fast to limiting the hours in which you eat. In the 20:4 fast, there are 20 hours of fasting and a four-hour window for eating. In the 16:8 (or 18:6) you eat in the specified timeframe and fast the rest. Of course, when you consider your hours of sleep as part of the total, that helps. Several small studies have shown success with fasting programs. Fasting may prolong your lifespan, as well as offer other health benefits. The problem? Fasting is hard to do for extended periods of time and can lead to extreme binge eating episodes when you stop. There are not any long-term studies on fasting and sustainable weight loss.

Expected weight loss from a fasting program ranges from as little as one to two pounds or up to 10 to 20 pounds, depending on how closely you follow the fasting program. As your body adapts to fasting, your appetite decreases and you burn calories more efficiently, which is good for your health. However, severe caloric restriction is not the answer, as all your organs—especially the brain—need critical nutrients to function.

We recommend intermittent fasting (IF). The easiest IF protocol to start with is the 14:10—fast for 14 hours and eat all meals within 10 hours. Make it a hard and fast rule: I will take my first bite at 8 AM and my last by 6 PM (or some combination thereof). Do not eat after 6 PM—just have water at night. This can be further modified to a shorter period of eating (fast 16 and eat 8) or even a shorter period of eating (fast 18 and eat 6).

Rules always work better than diets. IF can be hard to do, especially avoiding snacks like brownies, cookies, or chips at night (very tempting, as we know!). Eat appropriately-sized meals, consume no more than 1,800 to 2,000 calories for the day, and have only water at night. Sufficient sleep (at least seven hours per night) is critical to weight loss as well. Try the IF 14:10 and then you can shorten the eating interval to seven hours or even six. It is hard to go less—you feel like you're starving and may end up with low blood sugar. Every other day fasting or multiple days of fasting can be harmful to your body and are no more effective for weight loss than shorter fasts.

Take-Home Point

- Intermittent fasting does work for weight loss, and long-term success depends on your adherence. Give it a try!

Reflection Questions

1. Are your eating habits structured now?

2. Are you able to limit food intake for up to 14 hours? More?

CHAPTER 5

WHAT, WHEN AND HOW TO EAT

NUTRITIOUS EATING IS LIKE STANDING UP AND NOT falling down; it's all about balance. Keeping your balance in nutrition is to strive for a balance of carbohydrates, proteins and fats. Yes, that's what we said first; carbohydrates: the very carbs which many diets try to take away from you!

Well, let's talk about that. Some dieters have lost a lot of weight on low carb-high protein or fat diets, over the short-term. But nobody is offering any evidence of what the long-term effects of protein/fat-heavy, low carb diets are! However, the nutritional experts do know. The fact is, the body can survive almost any nutritional program inflicted upon it, be it starvation, or obesity—but the one thing it can't tolerate forever is an all-protein/fat diet. You don't need a nutritionist to tell you that sooner or later you need carbs to give you the energy, get the exercise you need, manage your weight, and stay well! Carbs are so vital that they should make up at least 50% of your diet—and come from the right sources.

Proteins and fats are just as important as carbs. If you get enough carbs, you require about 12–20% of what you eat in muscle-building proteins with the remainder coming from recommended fats and oils. In fact, more is not good. Less is worse. Realize that fats are not the cause of the excess flab on your body. Just the opposite. Fats in the "keeping your balance" nutrition plan are needed to make the carbs and proteins go to the right places and help you remove the flab.

When it comes to eating different types of food, our bodies respond differently depending on what we eat. You will probably find yourself with a sleepy feeling after eating carbohydrates. Proteins, however, make you feel more alert. That's why they're good to include at lunch and for a quick pick-me-up snack. Those peanut butter and jelly sandwiches we craved as kids turn out to be a good idea after all. Fats are what help make you feel satisfied or full, and that's why they need to be a part of meals as well.

Just as important as the balance is the timing, which means starting like you'd start anything else—at the beginning—with breakfast. Millions and millions of people employ the two lamest excuses in history: "I don't have time for breakfast" and 'I'm not hungry."

Of course they don't "have time" because they don't get up and do it. They may not be hungry because they stuffed themselves before bedtime to make up for the fact that they skipped breakfast yesterday and the day before that and that and that! And, by the way, don't fall for the nutrition bar scam, either. There are no substitutes for breakfast.

Timing means taking the time. One strong reason why you may not be hungry at breakfast time is because your tight schedule won't allow brief morning exercise, aerobics, jogging, or even a walk outside to work up an appetite. If you snatch a moment to grab a bite and stuff it down, you are not taking the time to enjoy the daily meal you need most. By eating too fast, you may be uncomfortable all day. Take time to prepare something you like, chew thoroughly, and enjoy every bite!

Now let's talk lunch. Ever watch a co-worker devour a submarine sandwich and try to talk at the same time? It even makes you ill, not to mention that you have no idea what they're saying. Others do without the midday meal altogether, surviving on coffee, soda, and sweets!

Many people rush to run errands after the workday and gorge themselves at night.

That evening meal should be your lightest. And make it relatively early. Remember the old adage to eat breakfast like a king, lunch like a prince, and supper like a pauper? You don't need an abundance of calories to sleep, because you're not burning calories so fast.

This is not to say you can't have a wholesome snack before you retire to bed, or a pick-me-up mid-morning or mid-afternoon for that matter. In fact, light snacks are a good idea, because you won't want to gorge at the nighttime meal.

Take-Home Points

- If you want to lose weight, you must eat.

- You cannot lose weight or manage your weight successfully if you don't eat when your body signals that it's hungry.

- You need to pace your eating—not just meals, but snacks too—to coincide with your activity level at various points during your day.

Reflection Questions

1. Try recording a few days of intake and observe how you're eating.

2. Are you going long periods of time during the day with very little or no nutrition intake?

3. What can you do to begin to add more food into your daily routine?

CHAPTER 6

WEIGHT LOSS AND WATER

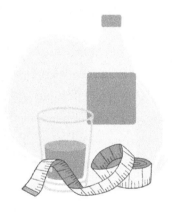

THERE'S A MIRACULOUS SUBSTANCE THAT CAN AID any fitness plan, is good for your skin, decreases your appetite, restores your energy, and lets you work and play harder. It's usually free and doesn't have a single calorie. Want some of this miracle elixir? Turn on your tap and get some good old H2O.

Sadly, in much of the world, clean drinking water is a luxury. But in developed countries, we're blessed with drinkable water in almost every city and town. But all too often, we go to the convenience store and spend $3 on a sugary, caffeinated drink that does nothing for us but add unnecessary calories.

Unless the drinking water in your region is heavily chlorinated or the pipes are bad, turning on the tap in your kitchen sink and filling up a glass is nearly as good as anything you can buy. If you don't like the taste of your tap water, there are numerous affordable water home filtration systems available.

The dirty little secret is that sometimes thirst registers as hunger: You think you're hungry, but you're just thirsty. Why does this matter? Because after you drink, you'll feel fuller, and you won't overeat.

If you drink a glass of water before you eat, you'll eat less. Doctors have known for a long time we simply don't ingest enough water, which leads to urinary tract infections, kidney stones, dehydration, headaches, fatigue, and a vast number of other symptoms. Don't wait until you're thirsty to drink—have at least 12 ounces of water every two hours while you're awake and at least a 12-ounce glass of water prior to eating. Drink water with your meals as well.

In a 2021 study published in the journal *Clinical Nutrition*, individuals who drank more water had a decrease in waist circumference after two years of follow-up.

Take-Home Point

- The simple act of drinking water decreases your appetite and limits the amount you'll eat, and will help you to lose weight.

Reflection Questions

1. Try recording your water intake for a few days. Are you hydrating your body?

2. Think about ways to increase your water intake if you find your intake is low.

CHAPTER 7

WHERE DID MY WAIST GO?

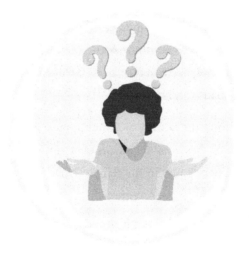

IF YOU'RE A FEMALE AND 40 OR OLDER, YOU'VE PROB-ably noticed your body has changed. Dropping weight is not as easy as it was during your teens, twenties or thirties. This is frustrating and begs the question, "What is happening to my body?"

The answer is simple: estrogen. Estrogen levels rise when women enter their teen years, marking the onset of puberty. Bodies change, and women develop hips, breasts, and waistlines, and begin to menstruate. Estrogen helps keep bones strong and helps store fat for childbearing

Women generally maintain this level of estrogen until perimenopause, the time leading up to menopause. Menopause is when a woman's menstrual cycles have stopped for a period of 12 months. Menopause begins at an average age of 51. During perimenopause, which typically lasts from four to eight years, estrogen levels once again begin to change. During perimenopause and menopause, estrogen levels drop and ovaries begin producing less. Just as we would not expect our bodies to return to a prepubescent shape after puberty, the same holds true on the other end of the scale: We can't expect our bodies to be the same as they were in our teens, twenties or thirties once we reach perimenopause and menopause.

Determining the start of perimenopause is not an exact science and is usually based on diagnosis of symptoms. Not all women experience perimenopause in the same way, however, typical symptoms include:

- Hot flashes

- Irregular menstrual cycle

- Increasing waistline

- Mood changes

- Sleep pattern changes

- Vaginal dryness

- Brain fog

- Constipation and bloating

- Elevation in cholesterol levels

In addition to a thicker waistline, women may notice more fat around the armpits and back. There may seem to be more fat and less muscle. All of these changes are real and part of perimenopause/ menopausal changes. And it means that you have to change your game plan.

The Centers for Disease Control and Prevention estimates the average lifespan for an American woman at 79 years, which means many women will live 30% to 40% of their lives in a post-menopausal state.

Keep in mind that estrogen is not the only hormone at play, but is one of the leading hormones behind some of these changes. The risk for developing osteopenia or osteoporosis increases during perimenopause/menopause, as does risk for heart disease and metabolic syndrome. All of these factors require change in our game plan. Following starvation-type diets, ketogenic-type diets or other trendy diets is now off the table. Perimenopausal/menopausal women have hearts, bones, brains, and muscles to take care of.

Another major process begins during this same time period. Called sarcopenia, it's the natural muscle wasting that takes place with the aging process. We can't stop it but we can slow it down by choosing our activities. We already know that metabolism is, in part, affected by percentage of muscle versus fat. Because we naturally lose muscle and gain percent body fat beginning in our forties, this directly impacts caloric consumption: You can't take in more than you can reasonably burn. We must ensure we have adequate energy to function. If we don't consume enough food for the liver to make the needed glucose, your body will break down its own lean muscle to produce it. The body breaks down muscle because it can't make glucose from body fat.

Take-Home Point

- While this chapter only touches on the many factors at play during perimenopause and menopause, it does shed light on what is happening in a woman's body and why the game plan requires changes.

Reflection Questions

1. Have you or are you experiencing any symptoms associated with perimenopause/menopause?

2. Have you noticed that you are carrying your weight differently?

3. Have you changed your weight-management techniques from your twenties and thirties?

CHAPTER 8

SELF-CARE

RESEARCH IS THE FOUNDATION FOR MANY THEORIES of self-care, and understanding the research is useful in planning a self-care program. Information about how a self-care approach was developed and why it works can help direct choices for a new season of self-care.

Learning how to assess information and whether you can trust it involves a minimum of five basic steps:

1. Ask who is conducting the research and if they have the required qualifications.

2. Determine if the research has been conducted on humans or only animals.

3. Discover who is funding the research.

4. Find out how many people participated in the study.

5. Determine if the research has been repeated and if it has been peer-reviewed.

Using these steps can boost confidence in incorporating a certain approach into a self-care routine.

As a starting point, these are some research-based self-care approaches we find trustworthy:

- **The Blue Zones**—The concept of blue zones grew out of the demographic work done by Dr. Gianni Pes and Michel Poulain, Ph.D., outlined in the *Journal of Experimental Gerontology*, identifying Sardinia as the region of the world with the highest concentration of male centenarians. Pes and Poulain drew concentric blue circles on the map highlighting these villages of extreme longevity and began to refer to this area inside the circle as the blue zone. Building on that demographic work, Dr. Dan Buettner pinpointed other longevity hotspots around the world and dubbed them blue zones: Okinawa, Japan; Sardinia, Italy; Nicoya, Costa Rica; Ikaria, Greece; and Loma Linda, California. www.bluezones.com

- **The works of Dr. Kenneth Cooper**—Dr. Kenneth H. Cooper, former Air Force Colonel, preventive medicine pioneer and "father of aerobics," introduced the concept of exercising in pursuit of good health when he launched the world-wide phenomenon aerobics in 1968. www.cooper aerobics.com/Cooper-Institute.aspx

- **The works of Dr. Andrew Weil**—Dr. Weil has devoted the past 30 years to developing, teaching, and educating others on the principles of integrative medicine. Dr. Weil is an internationally-recognized expert on integrative medicine, medicinal herbs, and mind-body interactions. The founder of Weil Lifestyle, LLC, a leading resource for integrative medicine education, information, products, and services, Dr. Weil combines a Harvard education and a lifetime of practicing integrative medicine to provide a unique approach to health care which encompasses body, mind, and spirit. www.drweil.com

- **The works of Dr. Wayne Dyer**—Dr. Dyer was an internationally renowned author and speaker in the fields of self-development and spiritual growth. Over the four decades of his career, he wrote more than 40 books, including 21 *New York Times* bestsellers. He created many audio and video programs and appeared on thousands of television and radio shows. www.drwaynedyer.com

- **Positive Psychology**—Positive psychology is a branch of psychology focused on the character strengths and behaviors that allow individuals to build a life of meaning and purpose: to move from surviving to flourishing. Theorists and researchers in the field have sought to identify the elements of a good life. They have also proposed and tested practices for improving life satisfaction and well-being. https://ppc.sas.upenn.edu/people/martin-ep-seligman A number other sites also have resources available.

- **MyPlate**—MyPlate.gov is your access point to the USDA's guidance on food and nutrition and is updated and managed by the USDA Center for Nutrition Policy and Promotion. This website helps users find what they need quickly and easily. www.MyPlate.gov

- **Omega Women's Leadership Center**—This Center offers an integrated approach to personal growth, leadership development, and social change. Whether you are a seasoned leader or beginning your leadership voyage, the Center's programs are designed for all who identify as women to strengthen their leadership so that we can help create a world that works—for everybody. www.eomega.org/womens-leadershipcenter/home

There are many approaches and practices of self-care that you can incorporate into your lifestyle. Rather than making a snap decision, review some well-documented practices to see what makes the most sense to you. You may also want to consult with a therapist or other health and wellness professionals to discuss and explore various options.

Take-Home Point

- When thinking about spiritual, psychological, and physical self-care practices you may want to try, it's important to review the research that supports their efficacy. By doing so, you are saying that your health is important and you're going to take it seriously. What you do today will impact the quality of your future years.

Reflection Questions

1. A feedback process you can use to improve self-care is the Start, Stop and Continue assessment. Briefly, ask yourself:

   - What do you need to START doing to take better care of yourself?

   - What do you need to STOP doing to take better care of yourself?

   - What do you need to CONTINUE doing to take better care of yourself?

CHAPTER 9

ASSEMBLING A HEALTHY SUPPORT TEAM

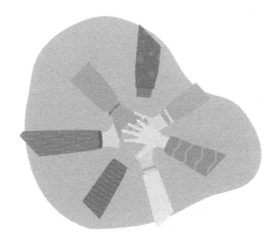

WHEN DECIDING TO FOCUS ON BETTER HEALTH, YOU need a support team. Social support from a partner, a loved one, family members, friends, and others is usually what comes to mind. Don't forget to include professionals such as doctors, dietitians/nutritionists, exercise professionals, and mental health providers. It is essential that you trust and connect with all of these individuals when you're making a major decision such as becoming healthier.

Your support team members should be:

- Trustworthy

- Honest

- Non-judgmental

- Knowledgeable in their fields

- Good listeners/communicators

- Empathetic

- People you feel comfortable with

You should:

- Stay in touch with them.

- Show your appreciation.

- Be available to them, if needed.

- Accept their assistance.

- Respect their limits.

- Know when it's time to change.

You should also consider other types of support that nurture and feed the spiritual aspects of your life, if applicable. Some individuals may look to spiritual readings and holy books as the basis of caring for body and mind. For example, there are hundreds of Bible verses that address taking care of your body: "Do you know that you are God's temple and that God's Spirit dwells in you? If anyone destroys God's temple, God will destroy him. For God's temple is holy, and you are that temple." (1 Corinthians 3:16–17). According to Jewish tradition, to take care of one's body is a mitzvah (a good deed). This mandate can be implied in the words "take heed to thyself and take care of your lives" (Deuteronomy 4:9). In the Qur'an, Allah has recommended that we "eat what is lawful and good in the Earth" (2:168). Further readings from these books and others can offer a sense of direction, instruction, and much-needed support to assist with your focus on heathier living.

Some practical suggestions for the day-to-day tasks of making a healthier you could include the following:

- Many of us find it helpful to exercise with others. If this is true for you, find an exercise buddy who is also focused on better health. Whether you are going to a gym or exercising at home, doing it with a supportive individual can make it fun and enjoyable.

- If you are more of an introvert and find it important to stay internally focused while exercising, being by yourself— whether at home or the gym—is the way for you to go.

- Make mealtime exciting. First decide what you need for yourself, at the specific time. Do I dine out by myself or with others? Whether it's making the meal or going out to dinner, decide what your preference is and follow it. Once you decide, put the pieces together for a wonderful experience. Eating is a time for total nourishment. If it's cooking at home, find a recipe that sounds good and try it out. Arrange the table and settings in a way that celebrates healthy eating.

Play some music that can be enjoyed by all and take your time to enjoy, enjoy, enjoy. If you've decided to go out for a meal, think about what your mind and body are looking for and pursue those eateries that offer it. Stay away from fast food since these selections will probably not move you in a healthy direction.

Your support system may change as you progress on your chosen path. It is important to keep in mind the reciprocal nature of support. By giving to others, you will receive and by supporting yourself you will create the reality of what you need.

Take-Home Point

- Within the next two days, take some time to reflect on what and who you want in your support system. Think about what you need and the various individuals who can offer assistance within that area.

Reflection Questions

1. How have I supported myself today?

2. How have I given to others and supported them?

3. Rather than doing what I have to do, what is it that I want to do?

CHAPTER 10

JUST BURN THE CALORIES OFF: THE EXERCISE MYTH

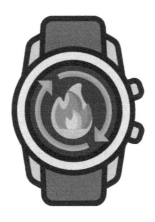

IT WOULD BE SO EASY IF WE COULD JUST BURN CALO-
ries off with exercise. Unfortunately, it doesn't work that way. While
exercise should be part of any weight loss program, vigorous exercise
without modifying intake is only good for slight weight loss at best.
That New Year's resolution to exercise and lose weight almost always
ends in frustration.

The problem really rests with metabolism. Vigorous exercise of any kind stimulates the release of cortisol, which in turn stimulates appetite. As a result, you tend to eat more just to maintain a baseline weight. Plus, it doesn't really matter what kind of exercise you do— high-intensity/short-interval workouts, marathon training, or vigorous weight-lifting—they all result in about the same weight loss. Your plan is to lose 10 pounds just by joining the gym doesn't work—you'll always lose more weight by also modifying your diet. The addition of exercise resets your metabolism to burn calories more efficiently.

So, the real focus becomes how to incorporate exercise into a weight loss program. Let's start with what you don't have to do:

1. You don't have to join a gym.

2. You don't need to hire a personal trainer.

3. You don't need to buy one of those fancy watches that tracks your calories and movement.

Here's what you need to do: Simply move. Exercise doesn't need to *feel* like exercise. Start by walking for 10 minutes a day, and every three days add another five minutes until you're walking for half an hour to 45 minutes five or six days a week. Incorporate the walk into your schedule and protect the time. Not a morning person? Walk on your lunch hour. Night owl? Walk after dinner. Meet up with a friend to add accountability.

You should also incorporate movement into your daily life at work, at home, or wherever you are. Here are our top 25 ways to start and keep moving:

1. take the stairs whenever you can.

2. choose the farthest parking space from the door

3. take a walk on your break

4. exercise before you go to work

5. garden

6. dance

7. walk over to talk to a coworker instead of emailing

8. rake

9. shovel

10. walk the dog

11. ride a bike

12. square dance

13. chop firewood

14. walk at the mall

15. scrub the kitchen and bathroom by hand

16. take the kids or the grandkids to the park and push them on the swings

17. snowshoe or ski

18. swim

19. find a YouTube exercise video that you enjoy

20. play miniature golf

21. walk the golf course

22. vacuum the entire house and re-arrange the furniture

23. get a stand-up desk at work and walk around when you take your phone calls

24. wash and wax your car

25. pick your own fruits and vegetables at a u-pick farm

Take-Home Point

- Exercise need not be exercise! Moving more in your daily life and beginning a walking program is a start.

Reflection Questions

1. How many steps do I take daily?

2. Is there a way that I can increase my steps without going to the gym?

CHAPTER 11

WHY AND HOW TO INCREASE THE RATE AT WHICH YOU BURN ENERGY

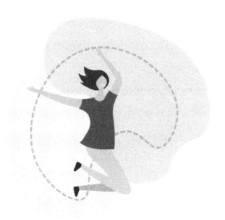

EVEN WHEN YOU'RE BEING A COUCH POTATO OR SLEEP-ing, your body is burning calories just to maintain your bodily functions and keep you alive. Metabolism is affected by three factors: eating, moving, and resting. The amount of energy your body uses just to break down and digest your food accounts for 5–10% of your caloric needs. Another 20–30% of the calories, or energy, you need goes to physical activity. But the most amazing statistic is the number of calories your body uses for breathing, beating your heart, and all the other things your organs do. A full 60–70% of all calories consumed goes just to keeping you alive, which is known as your "resting metabolic rate."

A key thing to note about how many calories you need just to exist is that your body requires more calories to maintain muscle than it does fat. So, one sure-fire way you can rev up your metabolism and lose weight is by increasing your lean muscle mass. It's also the reason why it's sometimes easier for men to lose weight than for women—men naturally have more lean muscle mass.

As you age, your body gradually loses muscle and develops more fat, an unfortunate process biologists call sarcopenia. Studies show that muscle loss can begin as early as your twenties. In addition, if you've been dieting to lose weight, chances are that you've been losing not only fat, but lean muscle as well. If you've been on starvation diets—1,200 calories a day or less—and/or high-protein/fat, low carbohydrate diets, most of your weight loss may come from lean muscle. When you gain back the weight you lost through dieting, it returns as fat, reducing your lean muscle mass even more.

Muscle is the only part of your body that actively metabolizes fat. The more active your lean muscle is, the more calories you burn throughout the day, whether you're running, sitting, or even sleeping. So if you want to lose weight, increasing your lean muscle mass and changing your body composition is the way to do it. Lean muscle is denser and weighs more that fat, so changes may not show up on the scale right away—another reason to stop obsessively weighing yourself. The good news is that muscle is about 22% smaller in size than fat, so what you can't tell by the scale, you can tell by the way that your clothes fit as you develop more lean muscle.

Pound for pound, you'll increase your metabolism and burn more calories by increasing your muscle-to-fat ratio. Nutrition experts have a rule of thumb for calculating the number of calories needed to maintain and lose weight: Multiply your weight by 15. That equals roughly the number of calories your body needs each day to maintain its current weight—and it's probably a figure much higher than most people believe.

Now multiply your weight by 10—that's roughly the amount of calories you can consume and still lose weight. Both of these figures take into account the fact that your body is composed of fat tissue, lean muscle, and, of course, fluids.

However, your body will burn more calories even at rest if you build up your lean muscle. It takes about two calories per day to maintain one pound of fat tissue, but it takes between 25 to 50 calories to maintain a pound of muscle. (Remember, by necessity, your body is composed of both, so don't try using these figures to calculate your calorie needs!) So, for example, if you put on 10 pounds of lean muscle while losing 10 pounds of fat, your weight would stay the same, but you would burn more calories every day, even while you're asleep.

The longest journey begins with the first step. (Always remember to get the all-clear from your primary care provider before beginning any exercise regimen.) Walk where you'd otherwise drive or ride. Climb stairs where you'd rather escalate or elevate. When you escalate, you're escalating your weight over the long run. When you take an elevator, you're not elevating your metabolism! So, whenever you can, walk. Just take a scenic, neighborly walk, a minimum of 20 minutes a day,

Step two is to step into a bicycle seat—a real bike or a stationary one—and get the wheels moving.

Step three is a dance step—or rather, many dance steps. Take lessons, or just call a partner and turn on the radio or a CD! Do whatever moves you, because pretty soon you'll discover that moving is more fun than you ever thought. You can also plant and tend a garden, or swim.

Formal exercise is satisfying and makes you feel better once you get into the habit. The purpose of formal exercise is to elevate the heart rate, i.e., burn more energy. How much formal exercise is enough? If you're just starting, start light with stretches and cardio. Breathe in as you prepare to make the effort and breathe out as you make the effort. You'll find yourself breathing deeper. You'll feel your heart beat faster.

You can do stretches and cardio every day of the week, but strive for a minimum of 30 minutes a day. As time goes on, some weight-bearing is good and, when you do start to include light weights, you still always start with stretches and cardio.

To boost your metabolism, eat at regular intervals throughout your day. As long as you eat meals and snacks when your body needs fuel, you'll keep the calorie-burning process going. By sating your appetite during those times of the day when you are most active, your body will store less energy as fat.

Take-Home Point

- If you want to burn more calories and increase your metabolism, aim to increase your muscle mass. Pound for pound, muscle burns more calories than fat.

Reflection Questions

1. Do I need to worry about how much lean muscle I have?

2. Is it getting harder to do certain physical movements like bending down and getting up?

3. Are my legs feeling weaker than they used to?

CHAPTER 12

THE METABOLISM FOLLY

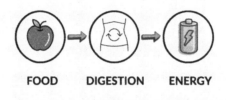

FOOD   DIGESTION   ENERGY

O VERWEIGHT PEOPLE OFTEN SAY "MY METABOLISM is too slow!" Many people think metabolism simply slows with aging. While there is some truth to this, it is not the cause of weight gain.

As we age, there are many different factors that influence metabolism, such as hormones, emotional state, and lifestyle. The reason drastic eating choices or radical dieting do not result in weight loss is because these changes slow metabolism and result in fewer calories burned.

Following an extreme calorie-restriction diet leads to three physiological changes:

1. You ignore hunger cues and overeat

2. Your body is deprived of food and wide mood swings spur you to eat more

3. Your body goes into a starvation state and feeds off itself

These three factors slow metabolism so much that your body hoards any calories consumed. So as backwards as it sounds, eating boosts metabolism.

Two other ways to positively impact metabolism are regular exercise and good sleep hygiene. We spend roughly a third of our lives sleeping. Unfortunately, for most of us, sleep is taken for granted and is not a priority. Yet numerous studies show that sufficient sleep has more to do with weight gain and loss than just about anything else: Less than seven hours of sleep per night causes weight gain.

So to lose weight, you need at least seven hours of sound sleep a night. This matters because we also know that sleep has a profound effect on something called heart rate variability (HRV), which indirectly measures a balance between your sympathetic and parasympathetic nervous systems, collectively called the autonomic nervous system (ANS). Relaxation techniques as well as various breathing exercises will also increase your HRV and balance your ANS, which is critical to maintaining good health and weight loss. HRV can be measured with a simple heart rate monitor (such as a heart rate band on polar.com) and using an app called Elite.

Most of the time, overweight people are in a hypersympathetic state with low heart rate variability, meaning they're constantly in a fight or flight state: Adrenaline is running fast, the engine is revved, and they eat more. The constant adrenaline rush causes a chronic inflammatory state, which is bad for your health. Inflammation leads to heart attacks, strokes, and weakens your body's immune system.

Take-Home Points

- Starvation is not a sound weight loss strategy.

- Adequate sleep is critical to lose weight and keeping it off.

- A balanced HRV is needed for weight loss and good health.

Reflection Questions

1. Do I get at least seven hours of sleep at night?

2. Do I turn off all electronics, including the TV, when I go to bed?

3. Is my room completely dark at night?

CHAPTER 13

TURNING THE CHURN INTO BURN

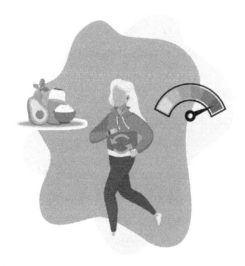

THERE *ARE* **ACTIVITIES YOU LIKE TO DO THAT YOU CAN** enjoy for exercise.

There's also another way to redefine physical activity. Even the experts are starting to take this into account in studies about fitness and disease. The category of exercise now includes all those things you do every day—walking, standing, climbing stairs, etc.—and adds them to the tally of how active you are and how many calories you've burned.

In this, our grandmothers and grandfathers had it all over us. Grandma cleaned, went shopping, lugged groceries and laundry up and down stairs. Instacart was not a thing. Grandpa would chop wood, wash cars by hand, mow the lawn pushing the lawnmower, not riding on it. Did they need to schedule a workout to get in shape? Ridiculous!

Yet, even in our computer age, there are still chores to do and routines that require physical exertion. The key, especially for the time-pressed, is to embrace these efforts as healthful movement and not as tedious work. The good news is that once you start looking into how much exercise you can get from the kinds of activities you take for granted, integrating exercise into your day doesn't seem so impossible after all. Even though you didn't start out with weight loss, cardio benefits, and increased muscle strength as a goal, you get to enjoy all those advantages as well. So, grab that hammer or dust mop and plunge right in.

Cleaning the house can burn between 200–300 calories an hour—more if you do it vigorously—as do feeding, dressing and taking care of your child, or repairing the plumbing. Ditto for raking leaves or sweeping the sidewalk or cleaning out the garage.

Like to dig in the dirt? Gardening can burn between 300–400 calories an hour. So can mowing the lawn with a push mower. Raking leaves burns between 200–350 calories an hour. Shoveling snow uses 300–500. Dress warmly, in moisture-wicking layers, for any cold-weather work or play. If you live or work on a farm, you have a big advantage. Planning a move? Carrying furniture and boxes of belongings back and forth to the truck, or up and down the stairs, can burn between 400–600 calories an hour.

You can increase the benefits of exercise by purposely making life a little tougher on yourself, too, by parking at the far end of lot for extra steps. Eliminate competition for that parking space closest to the entrance of the mega-mart. Even choosing to shop the super stores can provide you with some benefits as you browse the spacious miles of aisles. You can also use the stairs instead of the escalator or elevator. And, just for a change, take the dog out before he whines and scratches at the door.

The calculations need not stop once the chores are done. When you consider exercise, you should begin including those fun leisure pursuits you may not normally think of as effort. A simple game of darts will use 150–200 calories an hour, while ping-pong or table tennis will burn between 200–300. Horseback riding uses 200–300 calories an hour. How about badminton or golf? Both burn between 200–400, as does an hour of moderately-paced dancing. Ice fishing in the winter and stream fishing in the summer each burn 300–500, while ice skating gives you a great benefit at 400–600 calories per hour. Even something as easy as bowling or a friendly game of Frisbee can burn nearly 200 calories an hour. The idea is to start moving and to keep moving as much as possible, then watch the calories burn away.

Those who are overweight may feel at a disadvantage when it comes to exercise, but the truth is that the more you weigh, the more benefit you'll get because you'll burn more calories doing the same activity. And the more intense the activity, the greater the benefit for those who weigh more. For example, take riding a stationary bike with a moderate amount of effort. If you weigh 130 pounds, you'll burn approximately 413 calories an hour. At 155 pounds, you'll burn almost 500 calories, and if you weigh 190 pounds and ride at the same pace, you'll burn a whopping 600 calories an hour—nearly 200 more calories than a lighter person.

For moderate walking, at three miles per hour, a 130 pound person would burn 207 calories; at 155 pounds you'd burn 246, and at 190 pounds, you'd burn 302 calories, 100 calories more per hour. If swimming is your exercise of choice, the numbers are even better. For moderate-to-light freestyle laps, you'd burn 472 calories an hour if you weighed 130 pounds, 563 if you weighed 155 pounds and 690 if you weighed 190 pounds.

It's one more reason why, no matter what you weigh, you can benefit tremendously from starting even a simple, moderate exercise program and keeping at it.

Take-Home Point

• Obvious as it may seem, many people overlook the exercise benefits of routine chores and the pursuit of leisure. Anything that will get and keep you moving more can provide health benefits and even burn fat.

Reflection Questions

1. Are there ways you can increase your steps throughout the day?

2. What are some ways to increase steps while you are at home?

3. Are there some days that are not as busy as others?

4. Can you fit additional steps into your days that are less busy?

CHAPTER 14

WEIGHTS— NOT JUST FOR BODYBUILDERS

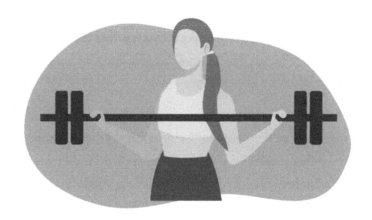

IMAGES OF OILED-DOWN, VEIN-POPPING, FLEXING bodybuilders aside, adding weight training to an exercise routine is one of the best ways to see faster results and change your metabolism by changing your body composition from one of mostly fat to mostly muscle. The current term is strength training, used interchangeably with weight training, and it's far and away the best addition to your overall fitness plan.

Strength training involves the use of resistance and weights, either with machines designed to work specific muscle groups efficiently, or with free weights. Either type will produce results. Best of all, only a modest amount of strength training is needed to achieve big benefits. In addition to the calories you burn while training and the lean muscle you build—which increases your metabolism—working with weights can produce "afterburn," increasing your metabolism for up to 15 hours after your workout. Aerobic exercise, while essential for cardiovascular health, doesn't keep the burn going as long. The main reason why building lean muscle burns more calories at a higher rate for longer is that during weight training, you're actually tearing down muscle. Later, when you're at rest, your body repairs the muscle by building it up. This uses more calories, which your body takes from its fat stores. This newly-formed muscle tissue also uses more calories, even at rest, so it's a win-win all around.

And, as you build more muscle, your body also builds more bone mass to support it. That's especially welcome news to older individuals concerned about losing bone mass to osteoporosis. And all this is true even with modest amounts of strength training. This kind of workout can be convenient for those with limited time to exercise. While the "30 minutes each day" rule for moderate activity holds true, your body reaps the best results from weight training if you work muscle groups every other day or every two days, giving your muscles resting time to repair in between.

Nearly any body type can benefit from the increased muscle tone developed through regular strength training.

Building lean muscle replaces what your body naturally loses through the aging process (which usually begins in your 40s) as well as any lean muscle you may have shed during past weight-loss attempts. Lean muscle burns fat and increases your metabolism even at rest. It increases strength and flexibility and is easy to add to a workout plan. Strength training, not diet fads and weight loss pills, should be the real health and fitness secret making headlines today.

Ever since strength training started gaining ground for its fat-burning and fitness potential, studies have been reporting other health benefits for a variety of age and population groups. A study done at Tufts University looked at knee pain in those over age 55. Half of those studied engaged in a home-based strength training program involving a set of exercises three times a week, while the other half concentrated solely on nutrition. Those who did the strength training reported a reduction in knee pain and better physical functioning overall, plus improvements in quality of life and self-sufficiency.

A study of men over age 75 was even more striking. The subjects started a strength training program due to weak muscles. They did eight-repetition power lifts just twice a week, adding more weight as they got stronger. At the end a year, their performance had improved at least five-fold, with some of the men lifting 600 pounds! Those who walked with the use of canes before beginning the program no longer needed them. Without question, strength training needs to be included in senior health programs along with exercise routines.

Take-Home Point

- Building lean muscle mass through simple weight training is the best overall way to boost your metabolism and manage your weight. But remember, you need both cardio activities such as walking and jogging along with strength training to be successful in keeping fit and burning fat.

Reflection Questions

1. Think about ways to increase your strength training during the day.

2. Think about chores that you do that can add to your strength training.

CHAPTER 15

THE PSYCHOLOGY OF IT ALL

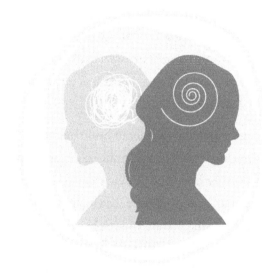

SINCE YOU'RE READING THIS BOOK, YOU'RE PROBABLY
somewhere on the journey of increasing the quality of your health.
It's key to better understand the resources you personally have at your
disposal to make the needed changes. Your thinking, behaviors, and

emotions are all part of this complex system we utilize daily to move throughout our world.

Let's look first at the thinking you use around weight. What are you saying to yourself about it? You may want to write your comments down to get a clearer picture. Are they critical statements like: "You've tried this before and it's never worked, so why are you trying again?" or "One more try at losing weight and one more time you won't lose, but you'll still be a loser."? Or are they affirming statements like, "I know you really want to get healthier and now is the time to make it happen!" or "This is the time to outline your personal strengths and put them into action to make you healthier."

What do you notice about the difference in these two sets of thoughts? The first statements are from an internal voice that is tired, defeated, and angry that the weight issue is still with you. They come from a place of weariness and uncertainty that yet another weight loss journey will be successful.

The second statements are about health and not about weight. These statements turn your focus to your health and how you feel— saying this is how your mind and body are right now and you're interested in making your "living machine" run better. You are not separate from your health; it is who you are and you have some choices to make about how you want your machine to run. Weight is measured by a number; it has a significance to you that may or may not be correct.

This is not about good or bad people, responsible or irresponsible people, or any other kind of divisive thought that causes you to feel judged and marginalized. This is about you knowing that you are ready to make choices that can assist you in becoming healthier. No judgment, no qualifying statement that you have been "bad" today because you ate a big piece of chocolate cake, just a reflection of "what do I need to do in the moment to be healthier in mind and body?"

Let's explore the inner voice a little more. If you decide to listen to it, what are the themes it usually uses with you? Realizing that this inner voice has been with you since birth, what it says about you has probably shaped much of how you feel about yourself and perhaps how you interact with the outer world. The inner voice has also been shaped by how people have interacted with you throughout your life. If you have constantly been criticized, the inner voice is probably demeaning and negative. If this is so, the issue may be how to change the themes.

A few thoughts on this: First, these statements are being made *to* you *by* you. In this situation, you are the speaker *and* the listener. Although the themes of these statements may have developed from how others treated you or what they've said about you in the past, you are repeating them to yourself and still listening to them. Why? What does it do for you to have such a critical, caustic inner voice? Some people say a critical inner voice motivates them. But do you want to spend time with someone who constantly negates and berates you, makes you doubt yourself and dismisses your strengths? You wouldn't spend time with someone else who did this, so don't do it to yourself.

Second, perhaps it's time to do a strengths assessment using an objective assessment instrument (this option prevents carrying forward negative themes that may persist if you complete a subjective self-assessment). There are several online assessments you can take to get at the core of your personal strengths. One highly recommended option is https://www.gallup.com/cliftonstrengths/en/252137/home.aspx which offers useful insights for self-discovery.

After completing the assessment, you may be able to create realistic, positive, encouraging themes for your inner voice, such as "As I better understand myself, I will continue to make better decisions for enhancing my health," and "I may make some mistakes as I work on increasing my quality of health, and when I do, I will learn from them and incorporate my new knowledge in moving forward."

Take-Home Point

- Take time each day to think about and reflect on the various components of your journey into a healthier lifestyle.

Reflection Questions

1. Take some time to think about the internal negative comments you make about yourself throughout the day.

2. If you find yourself feeling stuck about moving forward, take a few minutes to explore this following exercise, the 150% moment. Think back over your entire life and think about when you felt very excited, accomplished and just over the top...150%. What are the variables that made that moment in time so great for you? Are those variables present in your life today? If not, what needs to happen to make them present? Go for it.

3. If needed, create positive, realistic internal comments to combat the negatives comments that you already identified. Remember, sometimes you may need to fake it until you make it.

CHAPTER 16

SOMETIMES IT IS ALL IN YOUR HEAD

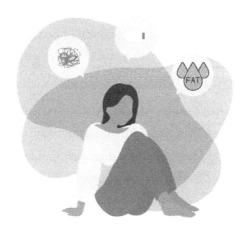

KNOWING WHAT TO EAT AND FINDING WAYS TO BE more active are only the beginning steps to greater health and fitness and, ultimately, to long-term weight management. Life is going to interfere: the best intentions are going to fall prey to stressful circumstances. What's more important than any one menu or workout plan are the strategies you'll choose in order to stick with a plan through days and times when nothing seems to go as planned.

The mental and emotional tools necessary for any successful health-enhancing program include:

- Psyching yourself up to stay on goal

- Identifying reasons why you may get in your own way

- Identifying pitfalls

- Recovering from setbacks without resorting to self-blame or the guilt trap

This starts with self-knowledge, which travels along the motivation path and leads to behavioral changes that result in success. You can't achieve your goals if you don't know what your goals are. Even if you carefully define exactly what you want to accomplish, you'll set yourself up for failure if you insist on perfection or define your acceptable outcomes too narrowly.

The first step is to figure out exactly what you're trying to achieve. Do you want to lose 10 pounds? Reduce your intake of high-fat foods or empty sweet calories? Avoid food binges? Get fitter or stronger? Reduce cholesterol? This is the part where many weight loss plans head down the road to failure before they even begin.

Studies on motivation and goal-setting have demonstrated specific strategies that can lead to successful outcomes with whatever approach that you decide to take.

Some of these strategies include the following:

- **Be realistic:** A 53-year-old woman who has battled obesity all her life is setting herself up for failure if she plans to lose 50 pounds for a special occasion that's three months away. A more realistic focus would be to target small weight loss increments over a longer period and begin to work on bringing out her own personal best features. Additionally, tuning out the cultural messages of youth-obsessed social media might be a part of her goal setting.

- **Be measurable:** Getting in shape means different things to different people at different ages. Cutting your fat intake by 5% is a measurable goal. So is working out for 30 minutes three times a week.

- **Start small and increase slowly:** Attempting to run a marathon if you've never even walked around the block is a sure setup for failure. The same is true for weight loss: If that special event is six weeks away, you'll only frustrate yourself if you want to lose 50 pounds by then. Small changes over longer periods of time will spell success.

- **Re-evaluate as you progress with your plan:** At 225 pounds, your calorie needs are greater than after you lose 30 pounds. Lifting five-pound weights for 15 reps may be a good starting point, and then you'll want to increase the intensity as you get stronger.

- **Be rewarded:** Celebrate your progress along the way by treating yourself to some special non-food luxury or reward.

- **Written down:** A goal that isn't written down is just a good idea. Writing out your goals and what you want to achieve and frequently reviewing them immeasurably increases your potential for success.

The Pace of Change

Often, when we discuss change, we tend to believe (or want to believe) that we are all in the same place of motivation for change. Whether we are discussing changes needed within a company, a school, politics, or a plan to become healthier, we may be at different stages.

To get a better understanding of how we change, let's look at two perspectives on change. The first views change as a circular, ongoing process that takes time, patience, and includes opportunities for new learnings along the way. It begins with a statement to others that you are about to move forward with your goal. We'll call this the "go for it" stage. You have been thinking about it, assembled a support system, believe that now is the time and need to move on it. So you move forward with an exercise program, a nutrition component, necessary spiritual supports and are on a roll. You feel motivated, look forward to each day's activities and things are generally looking good. Then, suddenly, you hit the "doldrums." You don't want to do anything except forget about your goal. You may feel like you've let everyone down, including yourself. Those little voices really do a job on your self-confidence. You want to avoid self-care and may even want to undermine any progress. Rather than practice any destructive behaviors you need to "cocoon." It is time to step back and learn more about yourself, relax, reflect and be nice to your wounded self and self-image. You reflect on what needs to be different and what learning can take place now so that you are ready to move forward when the time is right. During this time, it is important to remember that you are in charge if you choose to be. It is time to nurture yourself and learn how to move forward once again. It's time to get ready for another "go for it" stage.

Another perspective on change suggests that there are five stages, including pre-contemplation (you're unaware of a problem or the need for any change), contemplation (when you're thinking about making changes in the near future), preparation (when you actually plan to change), action (you're implementing a plan for change), and maintenance (you're continuing those actions over time). If you're in a pre-contemplation stage, you may need to be more aware of the risks of poor health resulting from an unhealthy diet and sedentary lifestyle. You can also be in two different stages simultaneously as it relates to different components of your goal. For example, you can be involved in a fitness program improving your health, and because of this, you may believe you can eat anything in the desired quantity because you'll exercise it off. In this example, being in two different stages will eventually undermine your entire quest. Developing a healthy lifestyle incorporates all components of your plan to reaching and maintaining your goal.

Take-Home Point

- Keeping one's mind body and spirit in balance takes focus, discipline and motivation. The result of this effort is the greater possibility of living your life healthier and to the fullest extent possible.

Reflection Questions

1. What are the specifics of your goal plan?

2. What stage of change are you in?

3. What else needs to happen for you to be ready to make the necessary changes to be healthier?

CHAPTER 17

IS YOUR GUT GETTING IN THE WAY OF YOUR WEIGHT MANAGEMENT?

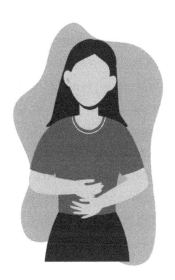

WE HAVE BEEN HEARING ABOUT PREBIOTICS AND probiotics for many years. We know that if we take an antibiotic, we need to eat yogurt to replace the "good" bacteria that the antibiotic eliminated while it was attacking the "bad" bacteria making us sick. How do those good bacteria get into the digestive tract, and what are they doing there?

Here's a partial answer—because researchers are still learning and studying it. Here's what we know so far:

- A microbiome—according to Joshua Lederberg (1915–2008), who coined the term—is "the ecological community of commensal, symbiotic, and pathogenic microorganisms that literally share our body space" (from "Ome Sweet'Omics—A Genealogical Treasury of Words," *Scientist*, 2001, Joshua Lederberg and AT McCray).

It is estimated that there are trillions of bacteria living on and in your body. Many are health-enhancing but, when out of balance, can become harmful. You also have more than just one microbiome—you have the microbiome of your gut, your skin, and your mouth. Interestingly, there are more bacteria cells than human cells in and on your body (National Institutes of Health news release, "NIH Human Microbiome Project defines normal bacterial makeup of the body: Genome sequencing creates first reference data for microbes living with healthy adults," June 13, 2012).

If there are so many bacteria, along with viruses, protozoa, and fungi, what are they doing? Here are a few interesting facts about your gut microbiome (from "20 Things you Didn't Know About the Human gut Microbiome," *The Journal of Cardiovascular Nursing*, November-December 2014 by Erin Ferranti, PhD, MPH, RN, et al.):

- It helps digest food, including the carbohydrates, proteins, and fats you eat.

- It helps make vitamins such as vitamin B-1, B-2, B-12 and K.

- It is essential for human development, immunity, and nutrition.

- When your gut's microbiome is out of balance, it is associated with autoimmune diseases such as diabetes, rheumatoid arthritis, muscular dystrophy, multiple sclerosis, and fibromyalgia.

- The gut microbiome is different between obese and lean twins.

There are foods that can help you better balance your gut's microbiome and make it more effective in keeping you healthy. There are the **probiotics**, otherwise known as bacteria, we mostly get from foods, especially fermented foods, including:

- Cereal

- Cheese

- Fermented milk drinks like kefir

- Kimchi (salted and fermented vegetables)

- Kombucha (fermented tea)

- Miso (fermented soybeans)

- Sauerkraut

- Tempeh (fermented soy)

- Yogurt

- Probiotic supplements (capsules, powders, tablets)

Now comes the important part. You likely grew up hearing "eat your fruits and vegetables." There's another reason to do so: For probiotics to live and thrive in your gut, you must feed them. What they like best is fiber, also known as *prebiotics*. Here are some of the foods that probiotics love for you to eat:

- Almonds

- Bananas

- Barley

- Berries

- Flax

- Greens

- Oatmeal

- Onions

- Walnuts

- Whole grains

Although there are other factors that impact the health of your gut microbiome, eating these foods regularly will help improve your overall state of health.

So, why is this important as you try to manage your weight? The latest research on microbiomes shows a relationship between the gut microbiome and weight.

- In a September 2021 news release from the American Society of Microbiology ("Do gut bacteria inhibit weight loss?"), Harvard Health Letter Editor-in-Chief Anthony L. Komaroff, MD, discusses how his opinion has changed over the past 10 years. He said that if he was asked 10 years ago whether the problem some people may have losing weight could be related to the types of bacteria living in their guts, he said he would have thought the people were crazy. He now notes that the research examining gut bacteria and its impact and mechanisms of promoting health has been rigorous. We now know that different bacteria help to break down our foods, and some types are better at it than others. If a person has a higher concentration of bacteria that is very effective at breaking down foods, it is possible that more of the nutrients and calories enter the bloodstream and tend to increase weight, as well as make it more difficult to lose weight.

- In the study *The Influence of the Gut Microbiome on Obesity in Adults and the Role of Probiotics, Prebiotics, and Symbiotics for Weight Loss* (from *Preventive Nutrition and Food Science,* June 30, 2020, Antoine Aoun et al) the researchers conducted secondary research, gathering studies from PubMed and Google Scholar. They learned that the gut microbiome has an impact on nutrient metabolism and energy expenditure. Additionally, different obesity treatments have been shown to change the gut microbiome, which leads to further exploration of the most effective treatments. They highlighted an improved understanding of how supplementation with prebiotics, probiotics and the combination of both, known as symbiotics, may alter the release of hormones, neurotransmitters, and inflammatory factors and possibly prevent food intake triggers that lead to weight gain. They conclude that further studies are needed to better understand which species of bacteria in the gut may affect weight gain and to learn more about appropriate dosing.

- In the study outlined in the journal article "Baseline Gut Metagenomic Functional Gene Signature Associated with Variable Weight Loss Responses following a Healthy Lifestyle Intervention in Humans" (American Society for Microbiology Journals, September 14, 2021, Christian Diener et al), the researchers look to find further information on why some people are able to lose weight more effectively than others. Their study identified specific "genetic signatures" in the gut microbiome that were predictive of weight loss response. Their study sample was small (105 participants) but allowed them to identify 31 functional genes. Their study adds to the growing literature that shows different types of bacteria in the gut microbiome can influence the success or failure of weight loss. The genes that allowed for more rapid bacterial growth were most closely associated with weight loss. It is thought that these microbes consume more of the nutrients in the gut, leaving less for the host individual.

- *Could gut bacteria microbes make you fat?* (from Emory University news release, "Scientists identify obesity-promoting metabolite from intestinal bacteria," January 7, 2022) looks at the influence of the gut microbiome on weight. We already know that no two people have identical microbiomes, including identical twins. We also know that your gut microbiome is influenced by your mother during birth, your diets, the environment and your lifestyle. In a pilot study (26 participants), Dr. Purna Kashyap, Associate Professor at the Mayo Clinic and head of its Gut Microbiome Laboratory, looked at the effect of a low-calorie diet on the effectiveness of the microbiome in digestion and making calories available to the host's body. While there was the appearance of one particular bacteria, called dialister, more frequently found in those dieters who lost fewer pounds, there is not enough evidence to suggest its role in preventing weight loss. As of yet, there is no clear picture of the differences in the microbiome between obese and lean individuals.

In another study (1,000 participants), researchers were able to create an algorithm which, based on individual gut microbiomes, can predict how blood sugar levels will react to different foods. This algorithm has been licensed to a start-up called Day Two. According to Dr. Kashyap, "The microbiome is changeable—we should be able to target it at multiple levels, which will each have an impact on treatment of obesity. There is no doubt the microbiome is a part of that solution."

Take-Home Point

- While there is still much to be learned about the gut microbiome and its influence on your health and weight, some things are becoming clearer. First, each of us has a different microbiome. Next, we each metabolize our foods differently. Lastly, eating fruits, vegetables, whole grains and nuts makes even more sense if you want to be healthy and manage your weight.

Reflection Questions

1. How can I change my diet to include more of these foods?

2. How will my family react to having our diets changed?

CHAPTER 18

DRUGS THAT MAKE YOU GAIN OR LOSE WEIGHT

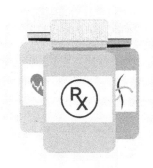

Medications That Make You Gain

Before you can lose weight, you should look at any medications you're taking: So many commonly-prescribed drugs cause weight gain. Regardless of the weight loss program you pursue, if you're taking some of these medications, you will have zero chance of success.

These commonly prescribed medications cause weight gain and can also make it difficult to lose weight:

- Anti-inflammatory medications like prednisone
- Antipsychotic medications like Abilify and Zyprexa
- Anti-seizure medications like Depakote
- Chronic pain medications like gabapentin
- Diabetes medications like insulin or glipizide
- Selective serotonin reuptake inhibitors, or SSRIs, like Celexa, Prozac, and Zoloft
- Tricyclic antidepressants like Elavil

Once a patient starts a medication, doctors are often loathe to stop them, especially if they think things are going well. If you're trying to lose weight, medications that make you gain weight are a losing proposition for sure, so complete a risk-versus-benefit analysis for yourself. Is the benefit of the medication worth the side effect like weight gain?

If you're taking one of these medications and are interested in stopping (if the medication is not required, like insulin), you should first speak to the health care provider who prescribed it; do not abruptly stop any medications without consulting your physician. Doses for drugs for chronic conditions can be adjusted down, and sometimes weight loss medications can be used with them.

Give Me the Magic Pill!

It seems like there is a medication for everything now: to lower blood pressure or cholesterol, boost mood, decrease anxiety, increase arousal. So why isn't there a miracle pill for weight loss?

Historically, a wide variety of medications have been used for weight loss, starting with amphetamines in the 1960s, leading to fen-phen (fenfluramine/phentermine) in the 1990s, which caused valvular heart disease and was subsequently pulled from the market.

Lifestyle modification is the gold standard for weight loss. When this approach fails you can try weight-loss medications. These are usually well-tolerated, effective, and safe. The question is when you should consider a medication, and which one is right for you.

Medications for weight loss are reserved for adults with a body mass index (BMI*) of greater than 30 or a BMI of greater than 27 and at least one other medical condition, such as high blood pressure, high cholesterol, heart disease, sleep apnea, or diabetes.

The primary challenge of weight-loss medications is that stopping results in weight gain, sometimes greater than your lost amount. However, weight-loss medications are a good way to jump-start your efforts when combined with diet and exercise. Let's discuss a few of

---

*   To calculate your BMI, multiply your height in inches by itself, divide your weight in pounds by your first number, and multiply the result by 703. If you'd rather skip the manual calculation, BMI calculators are available on a wide variety of reputable websites, including the Centers for Disease Control and Prevention (www.cdc.gov) and the National Institutes of Health (www.nhlbi.nih.gov).

the most commonly prescribed weight-loss medications that are safe, well-tolerated, and most importantly, effective.

Metabolism Boosters

Some weight loss drugs simply speed up metabolism to burn off calories. This class is known as sympathomimetic amines, or "legal speed." The most frequently prescribed is Qsymia, a combination of phentermine (an amphetamine) and an extended-release formulation of Topamax (an anti-seizure medication). You can lose up to 25 pounds over two years with continuous use. It is considered the most effective oral drug in achieving weight loss. Its major side effects include increased heart rate, elevated blood pressure, insomnia, and potential transient memory disturbance secondary to the Topamax. Qsymia has no long-term data on cardiovascular outcomes, but it appears to be safe

Appetite Suppressants—injectable

No doubt you've seen numerous ads on social media or TV about newer diabetes medications that promote weight loss. Known as GLP-1 receptor agonists, these injectable drugs were initially developed for diabetes and are now approved for weight management in patients without diabetes.

This class of drugs works by suppressing appetite. They are self-administered as weekly injections and are generally well tolerated. The two most commonly prescribed are liraglutide (Victoza) and semaglutide (Ozempic). (An oral form is available as a diabetes medication, but not for weight loss.)

In various placebo-controlled trials, these medications were effective in correcting weight loss by an average of 4 to 5%. In one trial, patients on Ozempic for 68 weeks achieved an average weight loss of about 30 pounds. The most common side effects are gastrointestinal-related, including diarrhea or constipation. Rare complications include pancreatitis and renal failure, and some studies have suggested that when these medications are used in higher doses for long periods of time they may cause gall bladder or liver disease.

Appetite Suppressants—oral

Metformin is an older diabetes medication effective for modest weight loss, anywhere from five to 10 pounds. This drug is not FDA-approved for weight loss but it's generic and inexpensive and is commonly used as medication for patients with pre-diabetes, or metabolic syndrome. While metformin is not as effective as other drugs in terms of overall weight loss, it's well tolerated and can curb appetite.

Other Medication Options

There are other medications for weight loss, but most have side effects that discourage patients from continuing. Orlistat is known for causing excessive diarrhea. Contrave is an opioid antagonist combined with naltrexone and Wellbutrin (bupropion), and its side effects include dry mouth, constipation, dizziness, nausea, vomiting, diarrhea and more, which is too many side effects for most people.

Another Option

A reversible surgical procedure, called a gastric aspiration device, decreases your intake and increases your sense of fullness. A small tube is inserted into your stomach during a 15-minute procedure. Connected to an external button on your abdomen, the device enables you to remove about 30% of consumed food discreetly into a toilet after eating (no doubt the grossest way to shed pounds). Left in place for about six months, the device can produce weight loss of up to 13% compared to controls.

Take-Home Points

- Some commonly-used prescription drugs make you gain weight and make it harder to shed pounds!

- Drugs for weight loss work, but the weight comes back when you stop them!

Reflection Questions

1. Are the medications you are taking making it harder for you to lose weight?

2. Are weight loss meds an option for you?

3. Have you asked your doctor about weight gain and the meds you are on?

CHAPTER 19

OBESITY IN OUR CHILDREN

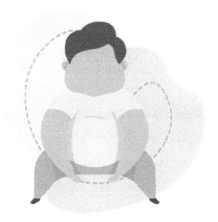

SOCIAL MEDIA AND TODAY'S WOKE CULTURE HAVE
taken a perilous path toward the normalization of unhealthy
weight for children and adolescents. That's not to say the rail-thin,
anorexic models of the past are the answer to marketing. But the pen-
dulum has swung too far in the opposite direction, with major brands
like Target and Kohl's regularly using overweight (plus-size) models

to sell clothes. Companies don't make this choice to be sensitive to overweight consumers but are instead responding to a market in which two-thirds of customers are overweight or obese.

Americans' sedentary lifestyles, reliance on processed foods, and even the changes in our daily routines caused by the COVID-19 pandemic have limited our society's overall weight control success. Rather than making an effort to educate the public about the benefits of a healthy lifestyle, millions of dollars are spent to normalize being overweight—while the percentage of diseases directly tied to weight continues to increase.

What's needed is a complete paradigm change towards health. We're not doing enough to promote healthy eating habits and physical activity in schools. One thing is for sure: Overweight children and adolescents become overweight adults.

Where to start? Numerous studies have shown that parents who practice healthy lifestyles have children who do the same. Begin with the following:

- Eat together as a family. This tradition has almost been lost in the age of travel sports or other activities that keep families running and turning to fast food multiple times per week.

- Plan meals. Unplanned meals are often pre-packaged and unhealthy.

- Don't let sports and other extracurricular activity control your lives. Family time is important and sitting at the table together is one of the few things most families do as a unit. Place a value on this.

- If you can't be home, that doesn't mean you can't plan a healthy meal to eat together on the road,.

- Eat healthier snacks—try carrots, celery, apples, and other fruits along with nuts.

- Encourage family walks, jogs, volleyball, soccer, ping-pong—anything that gets you moving.

- Live healthy and show your kids the value of eating healthier foods, avoiding junk, and exercising as part of your daily routine.

Take-Home Point

- Modeling healthy habits is easier said than done—you have to put in the work.

Reflection Questions

1. How committed am I to changing my lifestyle in order to help my children's health?

2. Do I need to sit with my family and discuss ways we can all start living healthier lives?

CHAPTER 20

WHEN ALL ELSE FAILS:
WHEN IS "THE KNIFE" THE ANSWER?

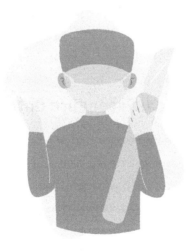

SOMETIMES WHEN ALL ELSE FAILS, WEIGHT LOSS surgery (also called bariatric or gastric surgery) might be the answer. You're eligible if you have:

- **Class 1 obesity**—a BMI of 30–34 and other conditions such as diabetes, and medical weight-loss therapies have been unhelpful.

- **Class 2 obesity**—a BMI of greater than 35 and at least one obesity-related condition such as high blood pressure, fatty liver, sleep apnea, arthritis, etc.

- **Class 3 obesity**—morbid obesity, or a BMI greater than 40.

If lifestyle changes and medications haven't worked or you can't tolerate them, surgery may be the answer. Weight loss surgery works: On average, patients lose up to 57 pounds and are at least five times more likely to have high blood pressure and cholesterol levels improve and for diabetes to completely resolve. Surgical weight loss patients may live up to 20 years longer. In the long term, no treatment for obesity is more effective than surgery.

Surgical Procedure Options

The two most commonly-performed procedures are laparoscopic sleeve gastrectomy and Roux-en-Y gastric bypass. The choice really depends on the expertise of the surgeon, your risks, and patient preference. The majority of weight-loss surgeries performed in the U.S. are sleeve gastrectomies, in which most of the stomach is removed and just a narrow "sleeve" remains. You feel full after eating less, which results in absorption of fewer calories. This in turn impacts the neuroendocrine system and the various hormones involved in weight gain.

The Roux-en-Y procedure is a bit more complicated—a small gastric pouch is created to pass food directly to the middle of the small intestine, which allows the absorption of fewer calories. These two procedures more or less dominate all weight-loss surgery done today. Older procedures such as gastric banding had high failure rates and are no longer used. The risk of perioperative mortality following weight-loss surgery is remarkably low (less than 1% of patients die during or after surgery), so these procedures are safe.

After surgery, patients should continue with lifestyle modifications such as regular exercise and avoiding binge eating. From a psychological standpoint, it's important for weight-loss surgery patients to remember the body will undergo a rapid metamorphosis, which can have profound self-image implications. Overeating can also be an addiction, and after a weight-loss surgery, some patients prone to addictive behaviors may turn to alcohol or drugs. Psychological support, through individual therapy and/or post-operative support group participation, is critical.

Weight loss surgery is not without complications: some 15% of patients may have early surgical complications such as bleeding, pulmonary embolism (a blood clot in a lung), or a vitamin/nutrition deficiency. For the rest of their lives, gastric surgery patients must take a multivitamin that includes calcium, iron, B12 and vitamin D.

Most weight-loss surgery patients will have excess fatty tissue, and about 20% choose to have body contouring surgery. Your surgeon will advise how long to wait for body contouring after your weight-loss surgery—typically after your expected maximum loss has been achieved and maintained for a certain period of time.

Sometimes weight gain can recur in patients who have weight-loss surgery, but this is typically related to overeating or a rare surgical failure. The vast majority of people who have weight loss surgery are happy with the results.

Weight-loss surgery isn't appropriate for everyone—those with severe heart disease, severe psychiatric problems, an active drug or alcohol addiction, or those whose weight issue has an endocrine cause such as Cushing's disease are not candidates.

Take-Home Point

- The bottom line: Weight-loss surgery is the answer for some patients. It's worth considering if you meet the criteria and all else has failed.

Reflection Questions

1. Do I think that surgery might be the answer for me?

2. Who do I need to talk to before making a decision?

3. What changes to my lifestyle do I need to make?

CHAPTER 21

TREAT THE ROOT CAUSE: YOU!

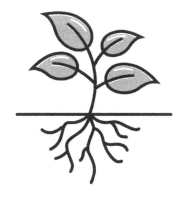

LOSING WEIGHT AND MAINTAINING IT IS A LIFELONG effort. 98% of diets fail because they treat the symptoms and not the underlying condition. Obesity is a chronic disease, much like high blood pressure, diabetes, kidney disease and many others. Unfortunately, medical professionals are often dismissive of patients who are overweight or obese. Doctors spend too much time blaming

RICHARD R. TERRY, HELEN E. BATTISTI, FRANCIS L. BATTISTI | **101** the patient for being overweight rather than offering proven treatments and strategies that work. They treat the symptom (your weight) with short-term strategies like diets that almost always fail. Ultimately, the chronic diseases progress and lead to an early death.

Diets don't work in the long-term because they're simply not physiologic—they don't mesh with the normal, natural process of your body. The Tomorrow's Weigh program offers a blueprint for success not only for weight loss but also for improved health. Wellness is not merely the absence of disease, but the overall well-being achieved by living the healthy lifestyle our program promotes.

Success with this program starts with setting some basic rules (and rules always work better than diets).

The Rules

1. Eat when you're hungry

2. Eat at regular intervals

3. Eat proper portion sizes

4. Exercise six days a week

5. Identify and avoid your trigger foods (what is it you can't stop eating?)

6. Consult your physician if think you qualify for weight loss medications or weight loss surgery

Let weight loss become the new symptom of your lifestyle change just as weight gain was the symptom of your old lifestyle—it sounds cheesy but it works. Our program offers a strategy that's proven successful in thousands of patients who have lost weight and kept it off, and you can do it, too. Weight loss will not happen fast. Gradual weight loss (a pound or two per week at most) will lead to a reset of your baseline weight. Be courageous, turn the page, and begin.

If you get frustrated along the way, online medical, nutritional and psychological support is available.

Take-Home Point

- Success in achieving and sustaining weight loss is not about dieting, but about lifestyle changes.

Reflection Questions

1. Now that you have completed the Tomorrow's Weigh book, what are the first lifestyle changes that you have made?

2. How will you sustain these changes in the upcoming year?

3. Which lifestyle change do you need to make next?

MODULE 1

INTRODUCTION

WELCOME! CONGRATULATIONS ON PICKING UP THE reins to your personal health. You've chosen the best possible course, and we are excited and looking forward to working with you as you achieve your personal goals.

This program will challenge you to release beliefs about dieting and embrace a healthier, more realistic approach to managing your weight and health. This will be difficult at times, and we encourage you to ask all questions you may have.

Housekeeping Chores

- Remember to plan at least one year to work through this program. A shorter timeframe will not provide you with long-term results.

- If life becomes chaotic and you find yourself not making the anticipated changes, DON'T QUIT! Too often, when we are doing well, we show up to do the work, and when we are not, we stay away. Do the opposite! If you're doing well and something comes up, maybe it's okay to miss a session. But if you are not doing well, that's when you need to get to your session the most! In other words, reach out to us!

- Be sure to complete each module before going on to the next. It is hard to be patient, but you will need the tools from each module to completely work through the next.

- Email us with any questions. The Tomorrow's Weigh program is pleased to partner with SpNOD (Specialized Nutritionist On Demand) to offer all our readers access to individual nutrition and lifestyle modification support. By partnering with SpNOD, all readers have access to 100% online support whenever you need it. You can chat online, call by phone, and video call. The SpNOD app is accessible in the App Store. You can also message Dr. Helen Battisti: at Helen.Battisti@spnod.com

- This program will address how, how much, when, and why to eat. We begin by looking at beliefs about eating and then move into planning your intake based on individual need. We'll look at portion sizes, and calorie, protein, fat, carbohydrate, and exercise needs, hurdles that get in the way, and more.

Before beginning, sit for a moment and close your eyes. See yourself deleting all the beliefs you have about eating, dieting, exercise and weight. Visualize your mind as a clean slate on which to build some new ideas. Gone is the notion of good and bad foods, that certain foods shouldn't be eaten, or that you're bad if you do eat them. Gone is the notion that you're supposed to diet all day and remain in control of eating at night. Gone is the notion that life begins once you reach your goal weight.

Picture yourself in this big empty room and begin building a whole new interior. Each time you hear yourself saying, "yes, but…" stop and ask yourself, "What am I finding difficult to accept and why?"

Let's Begin

Travel back to kindergarten. Go back to what we know to be true based on science.

Current fad diets ask you to believe that somehow, in a very short period of time, the human body's needs have changed. One year, we no longer require carbohydrates and then, lo and behold, the next year, we don't need fats. Then, before you know it, we don't need carbohydrates again. Whew…no wonder we're all confused about what to eat and just decide, "why not?" and leave for the buffet.

Think about it. The human body has not made any updates in at least 30,000 years. That means that it has required the same nutrients for all those years to keep bodies alive and healthy. Although modern technology is moving almost as fast as the speed of light, the human body is still in the Neanderthal era.

There are six basic nutrient groups: Carbohydrates, proteins, fats, vitamins, minerals, and water. In order to be healthy, the body needs all six of these nutrients in correct balance. It's just like a car, which needs gasoline, transmission fluid, brake fluid, oil, water, and antifreeze, but not in the same amounts. If the car doesn't have gas, but has all the rest, it doesn't matter…it's not going to run. Like a car, your body needs all its nutrients in the correct balance.

Remember, a healthy diet is not about food, it's about nutrient balance. The diet industry has placed all the focus on food and turned its back on nutrition. If you're seeking a healthy body and a healthy weight, then place your focus on balanced nutrition.

Most people approach changing their diet with the concept that they must get rid of "bad" foods and make up their new diets with "good" foods. Let's look at what most people consider "bad" and what most people consider "good."

Considered Bad	Considered Good
Desserts	Fruits
Chocolate	Vegetables
Ice cream	Chicken
Fast foods	Fish
Chips	Rice

The thought process is usually, "I am not going to eat any more of the bad foods. I am going to clean out my house and my office. From now on, I am going to eat only foods that are good for me!" This usually lasts one to four weeks. And then, little by little, the "bad" foods start making their way back into your diet. You become frustrated and finally throw in the towel, again.

Does it surprise you that this happens over and over again? It shouldn't, but if you believed the promises of the diet industry, you bought into the concept that you should be able to control your eating regardless of the situation.

There are two false assumptions in the previous paragraph. The first is that you should be able to avoid some of your most favorite foods forever, which is unrealistic. The most influential factor in how you eat is not your concern with health or weight, it's about taste. Taste will determine, in the long run, what you eat. If many of your favorite foods are on the "bad" list and you think you can avoid them indefinitely, you're setting yourself up to fail again. The second assumption is that foods are inherently good and bad.

Let's look at this more closely because this is a hard concept to give up. Think about going to the grocery store and buying a bag of "good" foods and a bag of "bad" foods, and then taking all those groceries to a chemistry lab. Once there, you perform an experiment to break each food down into its component nutrients, which is how foods labs determine the caloric and other label information. When you're done, all you will have are carbohydrates, proteins, fats, vitamins, minerals, and water…nothing else. This means that there is nothing nutritionally present in the "bad" foods that isn't found in the "good" foods. There is no such thing as a good or bad food. There is only balance, just like the car! You need fats and carbohydrates just as much as you need proteins and vitamins. It just needs to be balanced. This program will help you relearn what a balanced diet is. (Or maybe teach you for the first time.)

Can your diet be balanced if all you eat are sweets, chips, and fast foods? Of course not, but neither can it be balanced if you only eat fruits, vegetables, and whole grains. To begin a healthy change in your eating habits, you need to balance nutrients while satisfying your unique tastes.

Each nutrient has a deficiency line and almost all nutrients have an upper tolerance limit. If any nutrient is under- or over-consumed, there will ultimately be a negative outcome. For example, if you don't get enough iron in your diet, you will eventually become iron deficient and develop anemia because your body can't create iron. You have to consume it. On the other hand, if you have too much iron, you will develop hemochromatosis (iron overload) and become ill.

Think in terms of balance, not good or bad.

If you have no questions or "yes, but's," continue to the next module.

Does It Matter When I Eat?

Absolutely! Most of us have bought into the diet industry's message that you should be able to go all day and still be in control of your eating at the end of the day, which is completely unrealistic.

Think about how you usually feel when you come home at the end of the day. Do you come through the door and head straight to the cupboard or refrigerator? It's likely, especially if you were "good" all day and skipped breakfast and only had a light lunch.

Your body has certain built-in regulators that override the mind time and time again. Think about sleeping. Have you ever tried to stay awake for two days straight because you had so many things to finish? Do you find you can only go so far before your body says, "I have to sleep" even if your mind says "stay awake"? You will sleep regardless of how much you want to stay awake. And, you can't sleep for just five minutes, get up, and stay up for another 24 hours. Your body will keep you asleep for at least five to seven hours.

Let's look at another example: breathing. Can you hold your breath for five minutes? Of course not! It doesn't matter how conditioned you are, your body won't let you hold your breath for five minutes. If you *can* successfully hold your breath long enough, you will pass out and then begin to breathe again.

The same is true for eating. Your body needs calories to stay alive, just like it needs air and sleep. If you try to withhold calories, your body will drive you to get the calories, just like it does with sleep and breath. You can't be expected to eat next to nothing and stay in control…your body won't let you. You will binge eat.

Once and for all, most of us need to give up those 1,000 and 1,200 calorie diets **forever**!

Timing is everything if you expect to stay in control of your eating. Think about the last time you had your main meal mid-day. It may have been on a holiday or a weekend. Maybe lunch was served at 1 or 3 PM. Consider how hungry you were at 5 or 6 PM that night—probably not much. It's because, ironically, food is the number-one appetite suppressant. If you eat two-thirds of your daily intake by about 4 PM, you'll find your hunger declines as your day winds down. You'll make food choices according to your plan and feel better. You will also sleep better when your stomach is not full.

Step One

One of the first steps is to establish when you're going to eat, and then follow through with it. Think about your workweek and establish a time for breakfast, lunch and dinner. Then think about your weekend and do the same.

Write down the times and then list what you need to do in order to eat at those times. Do you have to plan your breakfast or make your lunch the night before? Do you need to have other people in your home take over some of your responsibilities to free up some time? Do you need to let co-workers know that you won't be available for meetings at lunch? Try to think of any hurdles that will prevent you from achieving this goal.

Don't worry about *what* you'll be eating yet, just get the timing down.

MEAL PLANNING

Review

How successful were you at following the times you established for your meals and snacks? How did you feel? Did you notice increased energy? Bloating? Sleepiness?

If you weren't able to adhere to the meal schedule you established, what got in your way? Are the obstacles movable? Does your schedule need to be modified?

Let's Begin!

Once your meal and snack times are established it will take continual effort to stay with them. You will be inclined to slip back to old eating habits when life gets chaotic. Keep working on it!

So, what should you eat at these times? Where to begin?

Let's start with the Food Guide Pyramid and explore the history of meal planning. The Food Guide Pyramid is a tool developed in the 1980s to help encourage balanced meal planning. It was born out of the Four Basic Food Groups developed by Fredrick J. Stare, MD, founder of the Nutrition Department at the Harvard School of Public Health.

There were different versions of the Food Guide Pyramid, including the Mediterranean Food Guide Pyramid, the Asian Food Guide Pyramid, and the Vegetarian Food Guide Pyramid, to name a few. The Food Guide Pyramid was updated in 2011 to the MyPlate to make it easier for people to follow. We will be working with the MyPlate. The USDA has created a website,www.myplate.gov that has a wealth of information.

As you can see there are five areas identified in MyPlate, including Fruits, Vegetables, Grains and Protein. The Dairy group sits off to the side.

In addition to the five food groups identified in MyPlate, fats are important to health and need to also be included. Fats provide the vehicle for fat-soluble vitamins and the essential fatty acids for proper cell development, which can't be made from anything else. There are different types of fats, including monounsaturated, polyunsaturated, and saturated. We all need at least three to four servings daily.

Finally, there are the discretionary calories which make up approximately 10% of your total daily calorie requirement. These discretionary calories are for foods that you love to eat such as sweets or chips.

Serving Sizes

Let's look closer at what constitutes a serving.

Grain Group

The grain group includes breads, cereals, bagels, starchy vegetables, crackers, and rice. Each serving in the grains group has approximately 80 calories, 15 grams of carbohydrates, 3 grams of protein, and a trace of fat (less than 1 gram). The serving size for each food in this group is based on these figures. For example, 1/3 cup of rice is a serving, which means it has 80 calories, 15 grams of carbohydrate, 3 grams of protein and a trace of fat. If you have 1 cup of rice then you have eaten approximately 240 calories, 45 grams of carbohydrate, 9 grams of protein and a trace of fat.

According to the Academy of Nutrition and Dietetics (AND) and the American Diabetic Association's (ADA) Meal Exchange Booklet, these are the grain group amounts that equal a serving:

Bread	1 slice	**Pasta**	1/3 cup
Bagel	¼ piece	**Rice**	1/3 cup
Cereal	½ cup	**Cooked cereal**	1/2 cup
Corn	½ cup	**Peas**	1/2 cup
Potato	1 small	**Mashed potatoes**	1/2 cup

Vegetable Group (Non-Starchy)

In the vegetable group, a serving is defined as an amount that contains approximately 25 calories, 5 grams of carbohydrates, 2 grams of protein, and a trace of fat.

Raw	1 cup
Cooked	½ cup
Juice	½ cup

Fruit Group

In the fruit group, a serving is an amount that contains approximately 60 calories and 15 grams of carbohydrates.

Raw	tennis-ball size (watch out for softballs!)
Canned	½ cup
Dried	¼ cup
Juice	½ cup

Dairy Group

In the dairy group, a serving contains approximately 90–150 calories depending on fat content, 12 grams of carbohydrate, 8 grams of protein, and 0–8 grams of fat.

Milk	1 cup
Yogurt	1 cup

Protein

In the protein group, a serving is defined as an amount that contains approximately 25–75 calories, 7 grams of protein, and 0–7 grams of fat.

Red Meat	1 ounce
Fish	1 ounce
Chicken	1 ounce
Tofu	½ cup
Beans	½ cup
Egg	1 whole
Egg Whites	2

Fat Group

In the fat group, a serving is contains approximately 45 calories and 5 grams of fat.

Monounsaturated

Olive Oil	1 teaspoon
Canola Oil	1 teaspoon
Almonds	6 each

Polyunsaturated

Corn Oil	1 teaspoon
Margarine	1 teaspoon
Walnuts	6 halves

Saturated

Butter	1 teaspoon
Lard	1 teaspoon
Shortening	1 teaspoon

The best place to look for the nutrition information in on the food label. Look at the calorie content and use that information to help you determine the portion appropriate for you.

Meal Planning

It's important to remember that everyone needs to consume the minimum servings from each group daily. This provides approximately 1,300–1,400 calories. Most individuals need to add onto this base number to bring you into the appropriate calorie range. Your weekly food record determines the range, which is why it's so important to accurately report your intake.

To start developing your meal plan, please find your *Meal Planning Work Sheet*. It is set up for three meals and snacks. Take out your weekly schedule and determine your schedule for the week and write in activities that will impact your meals.

For example, do you have an evening class, a late night at work, or have to get your children somewhere between 6 and 8 PM?

Next, starting with breakfast, write down what you plan to eat. For example: Two pieces of whole grain toast with low-fat peanut butter, one small banana, a cup of coffee and 4 ounces of orange juice. Remember, after the whole day is planned, the minimums from each food group should be represented. So, this example breakfast includes two grains, two fruits, and one fat. Now complete each breakfast for the rest of the week.

Complete this same exercise for your lunches.

Dinner is a little different, especially for busy evenings. Plan on quick meals or make-ahead meals for those nights and write in the meals you'll choose. For example, on the night you have an evening class, does a stir-fry work? That can be prepared in 20 minutes and provides a complete meal.

Write down all the protein sources you use, such as chicken, turkey, ham, beans, red meat, fish, or tofu. Write in the corner of each dinner block which protein source you'll use.

Rotate the protein sources, and then go back and decide which chicken dish you will make or purchase for a chicken day, which red meat dish you will make or purchase, etc.

At this point you should be looking at your meal planner and see that your breakfasts are filled in, your lunches are filled in and your dinner protein sources are identified. Let's finish your meal plans for this week by adding in grains, dairy, vegetables and fruits. Here it is important to remember color: You want meals to appeal to the eye as well as the mouth.

Let's work through a day—we'll use a chicken day as an example.

A baked chicken recipe will require an hour and fifteen minutes in the oven. Keep in mind that chicken is basically white, so pick other foods that have color. The grain group is also usually white, so it won't matter if you choose rice, potatoes, or pasta. You can jazz up the grain by cutting in a red or green pepper, or just serve the grain as-is.

The vegetable and fruit selection will really bring your meal to life. Let's pick a bright green broccoli, a bright orange carrot or maybe a fresh salad that incorporates the colors green, red, and yellow. For fruit, offer orange slices or a bunch of red grapes on the side of the plate, or maybe take a yogurt for your dairy and mix a fruit in. These options take only few minutes to prepare and will add brightness to your plate and nutrients to your body.

Now complete the rest of the week.

Finally, there are snacks. Go back and review your days and compare your snack options to the Food Guide Pyramid. What is missing? That should be your snack. If nothing is missing, you get to pick.

You have your mealtimes and meal plans for the week. Now you need groceries. Make a list of all the foods you don't have in stock and go shopping.

Working with a list will not only save you money, but also will limit the number of impulse buys, which grocery stores are designed to encourage.

Step Two

Plan your meals for one week. Make up your grocery list to be sure you have what you need.

Review your mealtimes and be sure they are appropriate for your week.

MODULE 3

REVIEW

HOW WAS YOUR WEEK? DID YOU STICK TO YOUR times? Did you follow your meal plan? Did you find yourself with more energy? What were the obstacles you experienced? What were your portion sizes? Did the portion sizes surprise you?

Let's Begin!

You are beginning to experience a new and healthier lifestyle. The changes will bring moments of new insight as well as moments of disappointment. The important point is never quitting—your future health depends on it.

Health is a life-long process that requires ongoing attention. It is a process that you work on every day, and nutrition is a key component.

While you continue to work on timing and meal planning, take the next step into increased activity.

Many factors play into Americans' decreased activity levels. Some of these factors include:

- community designs that limit ability to walk to school, work, and shopping

- increased technology

- increased fear of personal safety walking in their neighborhood

- increasing numbers of automobiles

- decreased biking/walking path availability

- elimination of physical education in some schools to meet budget goals

Sixty years ago, people used to cover approximately nine miles during daily activities. We now cover an average of three!

A key factor in maintaining your metabolism—the rate at which your body burns calories—is your percentage of lean muscle. As you become less active, your lean muscle begins to atrophy, or decrease. You will also notice decreased stamina, increased fatigue, and decreased strength and flexibility. Maintaining lean muscle is crucial to life-long health and weight management.

Take a closer look at your physical activity. Start with your daily routine: Are you at school or work most of the day? If you are at school, are you walking around a good part of the day, or is most of your time is spent sitting in class and reading? If you're at work, do you sit most of the day or are you up on your feet and moving?

The new guideline for all adults (age 18 years and up) is to be active beyond your usual daily activities for a total of 30 minutes every day. This can be done in a single block or throughout the day. If you have been inactive for a while, it is important to begin slowly and work up to the 30 minutes. If 30 minutes feels like a lot, think of it this way: Would 30 minutes of television be too much?

Let's look closer at the dynamic of exercise. There are two types: Aerobic and anaerobic, also known as cardio and strength.

Aerobic or cardio exercise targets the cardiovascular system and keeps the lungs, heart, and blood vessels intact. It also boosts metabolism and burns body fat. Anaerobic or strength exercise targets the muscles. Muscles will atrophy from disuse, as well as from the aging process. Strength training maintains lean muscle and boosts metabolism. These two forms of exercise produce the best results when combined.

Movement is not something you should do only for weight loss, but something that should be a habit just like brushing your teeth.

Before beginning any activity program, check with your primary care provider for a clean bill of health. Once that's in hand, another door has opened for you to increase your energy, improve sleep quality, improve your mood, and put a smile on your face!

We each have our own preferences for activity. Take time now to determine which type of exercise you prefer. You may want to begin working with a personal trainer to establish a program tailored to your needs, limitations, and goals. Or you may want to begin with walking in your neighborhood. The important thing is to start moving. If weather is a limitation in your area, check out the open times at area workout facilities, such as the local Y, high school, or college (many schools have a community access option). Exercise facilities with membership options are readily available throughout the country.

Please go to your Activity Record in the Tool Section and begin tracking your progress, which you will continue to assess as we proceed.

Take a few minutes to explore any hurdles that have taken you off-track in the past and those that might sideline you now and in the future. Excuses for not moving include: I don't have time; it's too expensive; I don't have anyone to go with; I have bad ankles/knees/back; the weather is awful; I'm just too tired. Remember, where there is a will there is always a way. Take a moment and write down your current excuses. Look at them. Can you think of solutions?

MODULE 4

TRIGGERS AND EATING CUES

Review

How are you doing with your recording and meal planning? Now that your plan is in full swing, are you finding that you're slipping back into old habits? Are you forgetting to go grocery shopping on a regular basis? Are you packing "meals on the run?"

How are you feeling after beginning your exercise routine? Are you enjoying the exercise? Do you have a partner, or do you prefer to exercise alone?

Let's Begin!

Remember that there are no "good" or "bad" foods. There are only the six nutrients—carbohydrates, proteins, fats, vitamins, minerals, and water—that comprise all food. When taken to a chemistry lab and closely examined, there is nothing lurking in certain foods that will undermine your efforts in achieving good health.

Trigger Foods

You may find that if a certain food is in the house, it calls your name continually until it's gone. You usually cannot stop eating these foods at the point you mean to. They are almost exclusively carbohydrates, such as potato chips, corn chips, ice cream, bread, cookies, pie, or cake. These are called trigger foods. They are not good or bad, but rather particular foods to which you are sensitive. These foods are unique to you. It is important for you to determine if you have trigger foods and, if so, recognize them and the effect they have.

Take a moment to think about your trigger foods. Make a list so that you are aware of them. If you don't have any trigger foods, ask a friend if they do and discuss them.

My Trigger Foods

_____

_____

_____

Usually, we buy trigger foods under the guise of having these foods available for family or friends if they drop by. You may see these foods on sale or visit a certain store where you know they're sold. This is all very noble, but it is important to face your trigger foods and realize that you need to stop buying them and bringing them into your home if they prevent you from managing your weight or achieving your health goals.

Managing weight means that you can't eat what you want, when you want, in the quantity you want. Managing weight means that you plan your meals, practice portion control and generally eat at the same time each day.

Trigger foods are usually your favorites. Managing weight means that you will no longer be able to bring trigger foods freely into your environment, unless you have every intention of consuming all of them. Don't keep these foods around for family or friends. You need to remove trigger foods from your home.

Does this mean that you can never have them again? No. What it does mean is that you must purchase these foods when you're out. You will need to purchase a predetermined amount to eat and enjoy before returning home.

For example, if you find you can't have freshly-baked chocolate chip cookies in the house because you will eat them all, it's important for you to stop making them. Do you have to stop eating them? Absolutely not, but you should go to a bakery, purchase a certain amount, and then eat them. When you are eating them, focus on your eating and enjoy the experience. Too often you half-notice you're eating and half-try to distract yourself because you feel guilty. There is no guilt in eating. You can't stay alive unless you eat!

Behavior Maps

When trying to make your way to a new location, you consult a map. Behaviors make a map that frequently led you to the same destination time and time again. Let's look at an example given by a past student.

Kate comes home from school/work each day at about 5:30 PM. She has two children active in sports. Depending on the evening, Kate usually must make dinner, get the children to their activities and home again. She also must be sure they complete their homework, bathe, and have clothes ready for the next day. Bedtime is at 9 PM. Once the children are in bed, Kate cleans up around the house, gets things ready for morning, and then sits down to begin her own homework. Once in her favorite chair, Kate's thoughts frequently turn to what's available to eat in the kitchen. She usually finds herself eating while doing homework, right before going to bed. Kate wakes up the next morning and tells herself she won't eat that late again, but it happens over and over.

Let's make a map of Kate's trip through the evening.

Arrives Home — Fixes Dinner — Helps With Homework —
Everyone To Bed — Sits Down

Make your own map. Do you find that you make the same trip each day and end up eating when you didn't intend to? Once you observe your map, you can re-route your trip. In Kate's case, her eating had become a reward for completing all her jobs and chores. Her eating was part of de-stressing. Once she saw the trip she made most evenings, she realized she could re-route: She started going into another room at night, after all her work was done, to begin her homework. She found that by moving into another room, it was easier to stop her nighttime eating. Think about other ways you can reach your destination that don't involve eating.

Step Four

Complete your trigger list and recognize the need to keep these foods out of your home.

Draw a behavior map of your usual routine and see if you can discover any set behaviors that lead to problem destinations.

MODULE 5

REVIEW

L IFESTYLE CHANGES TAKE A LIFETIME TO PERFECT. Don't get discouraged if you discover that changes you put in place a few weeks ago have somehow disappeared. Let's take a minute to review where you are and what you've put into action.

Ask yourself these questions:

- Are you eating two-thirds of your total food intake by 4 PM?

- Are you remembering to have appropriate snacks on hand for the morning and afternoon?

- Are you sticking with your exercise routine? If it isn't working, have you tried something new?

- Have you made a list of trigger foods and realized the need to control when and where you eat these foods?

- Have you made maps of trips you take that lead you into unplanned eating?

Before You Begin

You've chosen the Tomorrow's Weigh program, so it's apparent that you're working to become healthier. It can be difficult to maintain a healthy lifestyle with all the demands on your time. Remember to take it one step at a time. Go back and read your answer to the first discussion question.

In this module, we'll cover a wealth of information. Some will be useful to you and some won't—don't try to tackle too many changes at once.

Here's are two simple formulas to determine your calorie needs:

- **To maintain weight:** Multiply your weight by 15.

- **To lose weight:** Multiply your weight by 10. As your weight decreases, check in on your calorie number by multiplying your new weight by 10.

Keep up the great work!

Let's Begin

Going to the grocery store requires reading food labels, which give you the information needed to choose foods and beverages wisely. Go to your kitchen and pick a food with a food label and refer to it during this module.

Portion Size

The first label item to review is portion size, which reflects all the nutrition information. It is not necessarily the same amounts noted on the food pyramid. Also pay attention to the number of servings per package.

Calories

The next item is calories, a number that's helpful when determining your overall caloric intake—too often you consume larger amounts than you realize. Calories derived from fats are usually the grams of fat times nine.

Total Fat

Next on the label is the total fat. Fats should comprise 25–35% of a healthy diet's total daily calories, up from the previous recommendation of 30%. The majority of your fats should be monounsaturated, which is found in olive oil, canola oil, peanut oil, almonds, avocados, and walnuts. Saturated fat, which is primarily from animals, should be minimized and should make up no more than 10% of your total daily calories.

To determine this, multiply your total daily calories consumed by 0.10. For example, if you are losing weight and consuming approximately 1,800 calories, then 1,800 x 0.10 = 180 calories. Then, because all the information on the food label is in grams (g) or milligrams (mg), divide by 9 (because there are 9 calories per gram of fat). Therefore, the total saturated fats each day = 20 grams. Try to determine the amount of saturated fat you should consume. If you have high cholesterol or a family history of heart disease, limit your saturated fat to 7% of your total daily calories.

Sodium

Next is sodium. This number is always represented in milligrams (mg), so it's not unusual to wonder how much you should be eating. A no added salt (NAS) diet provides approximately 1,110–3,000 mg of sodium a day. Use this number when assessing the amount of sodium in your diet. If you have high blood pressure or a family history of heart disease, you will want to keep your daily sodium intake in this range.

Total Carbohydrates, Fiber, Sugar, and Added Sugar

Next are total carbohydrates, fiber, sugar, and added sugar. There is a lot of confusing information regarding the amount and type of carbohydrates required: The current recommendation is 45–60% of total calories. Carbohydrates are found in the grain, fruit, dairy, and vegetable food groups. Carbohydrates are also present in sweets and other snack foods. The following table shows where carbohydrates, proteins and fats are found in your diet:

	Carbohydrate	Protein	Fats
Grain	15g	3g	0–1g
Fruit	15g	0g	0g
Vegetable	5g	2g	0g
Dairy	12g	8g	0–8g
Meat	0g	7g	0–8g
Fat	0g	0g	5g

When determining the amount of carbohydrates in your diet, ask yourself:

- Do I have a family history of diabetes, or do I have diabetes?

If yes, you will want to keep total carbohydrates between 45–50% of calories, unless you are currently an athlete.

- Do I participate in physical activity every day?

If yes, you will want to keep total carbohydrates between 55–60% of calories.

If you do not have diabetes in your family and you are not physically active, you will want to keep total carbohydrates at 50–55% of calories.

To determine the amount of carbohydrates you should consume daily, let's use the same 1,800-calorie example we used in determining fats. Take 1,800 calories and multiply by 0.50 for 50% of calories. 1,800 x 0.50 = 900 calories. Now divide this number by 4, because there are 4 calories per gram of carbohydrate. 900/4 = 225 g. Try it with your calorie range.

Simple sugar, including added sugar, should not exceed 10%, is calculated the same way, and is part of the total carbohydrate amount. 1,800 calories x 0.10 = 180 divided by 4 = 45 g. Therefore, of the total 225 g of carbohydrates a day, 45 can be from simple and added sugar.

Fiber should be between 20–35 g each day. Fiber has been shown to help maintain regularity and blood sugar levels, lower cholesterol, help you feel fuller longer, and possibly decrease the risk of gastrointestinal cancer.

Protein

Protein needs should comprise 12–20% of calories. It is calculated the same way. Using 1,800 calories as an example, multiply 1,800 by 0.12 and 0.20.

1,800 x 0.12 = 216/4 calories per gram = 54 g.

1,800 x 0.20 = 360/4 calories per gram = 90 g.

Like the carbohydrate, there are 4 calories per gram of protein. Consuming too much or too little protein can have negative effects on your health.

Using the information on the food label can be very helpful when balancing your diet. If you have further questions, please email us.

Step Five

Now you must determine the balance of carbohydrates, proteins, and fats in your diet based on your total daily caloric needs. This will maintain a balance that can help prevent heart disease, diabetes, certain forms of cancer, high blood pressure, and obesity.

MODULE 6

T'S WEEK SIX AND YOUR MOTIVATION FOR MAKING
some of these major lifestyle changes may be slowing down, and
your initial motivation may start to wane. It is important to realize
that a change in motivational level is normal. Now is the time, however, to once again decide what's moving you toward making healthy
lifestyle changes.

Motivation is a complex process that has been studied and pon-
dered over the ages. Valuable related principles include the facts that:

- motivation is a process that evolves for each of us

- the same thing does not motivate everyone

- what motivates us today may change tomorrow, based on
  internal and external competing forces and life experiences

Let's Begin

Let's get back to looking at your present state of motivation. If you're currently following your plan for change and are on the mark for moving forward, stick with your process. If you are struggling or have stopped completely, now is the time to step back and look at your motivating factors.

It's important to remember that you've reached this point. By deciding to read this module, you still are motivated to making a change in your health status or completing this course! Use this opportunity to explore what's needed to keep your process moving forward.

Your level of commitment to staying with the process is the key to change. The spark for commitment is a clear, compelling vision of what you want to create for yourself. Take a few minutes and write down the vision of health you want for yourself.

The journey to health is not always a straight line. Health comes at different times and from different directions, and continuous forward motion is the key. Ask yourself these questions and think about your answers:

- What have I learned about my motivational qualities at this point in the process?

- Am I more internally motivated [I believe taking the necessary steps to being healthy is imperative] or am I more externally motivated [the way I look is the most important result of being healthy]?

- Do I need to team up with another individual or a group to receive and give support with changes?

- What were the barriers that I allowed to distract me from my original commitment?

- Are the barriers internal or external? What do I have to modify in my life to move beyond these barriers?

- Am I worth recommitting myself to a healthy lifestyle?

- Am I ready to recommit myself to the necessary changes?

- What is my revised plan for moving forward?

- What do I need to start, stop, and/or continue doing?

Remember, the key to commitment is a clear and compelling vision of what you want to create for your life. The future is not static: It is a place you create with your mind, then your heart, and then with your actions and behaviors.

Cycle of Motivation: Action

Motivation has been described as a cycle composed of three chambers. The first chamber is action. In the action chamber, you feel in control and like you're moving toward your goal. It feels like nothing can stop you, and it's exhilarating! But then, as it always does, the action chamber ends. How many times have you started something with 100% commitment and excitement only to find later that you lost it?

Cycle of Motivation: Cocoon

The truth is, you didn't really lose anything. The end of the action chamber brings you to the second chamber—the cocoon. In this chamber, you just don't want to do it anymore. "It" can be meal planning, homework, going to the gym, etc. This is the chamber in which most people think they have lost it.

It's similar to failing a test in school. You start your education in kindergarten and make your way through to senior year in high school. Let's say that in first grade, you fail a spelling test. Does that mean that you have to go back to kindergarten and start again? No—it just means you have to change your study habits a little. If you fail your math test in second grade, does that mean that you have to go back to kindergarten and start again? Absolutely not!

Cycle of Motivation: Planning

Well, the same is true with motivation. Moving through the action chamber to the cocoon chamber is a normal process. You will remain there for a while, but if you have a clear vision of where you are going and you keep your eyes on it, you'll move into chamber three—the planning chamber. This is where you look at what you were doing and begin to make changes. Let's use the example of exercise and say that you have been going to the gym all winter. It's working well until suddenly, one day, you come out of class and find that you just don't want to go to the gym anymore. You may find it hard to get there day after day and you are sure that you've lost it again. You may be arguing with yourself for a month or so when suddenly, you notice that the weather is warming up and you want to be outside.

You realize you don't want to be at the gym when the weather is nice. Now you are moving again and entering the planning chamber.

In the planning chamber, you decide what's working and what isn't. You explore other alternatives to the gym. You may remember that you used to enjoy riding your bike. You may need to get your bike out and see if it needs a tune-up, or maybe you just need to find the bike rack for your car and head to a park or trail to ride. Once your plan is in place, you are entering the action chamber again.

If you pay attention, you'll find this cycle holds true with most changes you're working on. It's important to remember you haven't *lost* anything and you are certainly not back at the beginning. Stay focused and remember that you only fail if you quit.

MODULE 7

CARBOHYDRATES AND YOU

HAVE YOU STARTED TO NOTICE THAT YOUR LIFESTYLE
is changing? Are the new habits you've been working on beginning to feel familiar? Now can be a very important time in your efforts
to make your changes permanent. Look at the goals you set at the start
of this program. Have you met some of those goals already?

Let's Begin

Let's review the information that we read in Module 5 about
carbohydrates.

There's a lot of confusing information regarding the amount
and type of carbohydrates required: The current recommendation is
45–60% of total calories. Carbohydrates are found in the grain, fruit,
dairy, and vegetable food groups. Carbohydrates are also present in
sweets and other snack foods. The following table shows where the
carbohydrates, proteins, and fats are found in your diet:

	Carbohydrate	Protein	Fat
Grain	15g	3g	0–1g
Fruit	15g	0g	0g
Vegetable	5g	2g	0g
Dairy	12g	8g	0–8g
Meat	0g	7g	0–8g
Fat	0g	0g	5g

When determining the amount of carbohydrates in your diet, ask yourself:

- Do I have a family history of diabetes, or do I have diabetes?

If yes, you will want to keep total carbohydrates between 45–50% of calories, unless you are currently an athlete.

- Do I participate in physical activity every day?

If yes, you will want to keep total carbohydrates between 55–60% of calories.

If you do not have diabetes in your family and you are not physically active, you will want to keep total carbohydrates at 50–55% of calories.

To determine the amount of carbohydrates you should consume daily, let's use the same 1,800 calorie example we used in determining fats. Take 1,800 calories and multiply by 0.50 for 50% of calories. 1,800 x 0.50 = 900 calories. Now divide this number by 4, because there are 4 calories per gram of carbohydrate. 900/4 = 225 g. Try it with your calorie range.

Simple sugar should not exceed 10% and is calculated the same way, and is part of the total carbohydrate amount. 1,800 calories x 0.10 = 180 divided by 4 = 45 g. Therefore, of the total 225 g of carbohydrates a day, 45 can be from simple sugar.

Fiber should range from 20–35 g each day. Fiber has been shown to help maintain regularity and blood sugar levels, lower cholesterol, help you feel fuller longer, and possibly decrease the risk of gastrointestinal cancer.

Carbohydrates have numerous tasks in the body. They are the primary fuel (blood sugar/glucose) for the body. Without carbohydrates, the body breaks down internal protein to make the necessary fuel, and your kidneys dispose of the nitrogen waste that results.

An athlete, or anyone who exercises on most days, requires even more carbohydrates. Your body stores carbohydrates as glycogen—required for the production of energy—in the muscles and liver. If your glycogen falls too low due to an unbalanced diet, you'll experience early muscle fatigue.

To determine the amount of carbohydrates you need daily, determine your daily caloric needs. Again, if you are trying to maintain your weight, multiply your weight by 15. If you are trying to lose weight, multiply your weight by 10. For weight loss, as your weight goes down, so should your calories.

Please determine your proper amount of daily carbohydrates and compare to the two days of intake that you enter for this week.

Emotional Eating

Some individuals use carbohydrates—chips, cookies, ice cream, or bread—when feeling emotions like stress. Consumption of carbohydrates makes you feel groggy or sleepy and can also quiet the unpleasant emotion. But it's temporary and often has the side effect of weight gain.

Review

Balancing your diet is about balancing your unique nutrient needs. There are as many right answers to a balanced diet as there are people. At the beginning of these modules, you started examining your diet with the MyPlate tool to help organize your nutrients. Now you're looking at the nutrient groups that make up the food groups. Last week you looked closer at the total carbohydrates in your diet and determined how much you need and how much you're consuming. This week you'll look closer at the protein in your diet.

Before You Begin

Let's dive deeper into the discussion about carbohydrates. Sugar is listed on the food label under total carbohydrates. This represents the grams of simple sugar found in the referenced serving size. This can get confusing: A simple sugar is technically called a monosaccharide and disaccharide. A complex carbohydrate is called a polysaccharide.

Some of the most common simple sugars that you see on food labels include:

Table sugar:	Sucrose
Fruit sugar:	Fructose
Milk sugar:	Lactose

When looking at the grams of sugar on the label, remember that it may not be sucrose. For example, fruit is 100% carbohydrate and is fructose or a simple sugar. If you have a question about the sugar, look at the ingredients listed and search for added sugar. If the product is 100% juice you won't see added sugar. The sugar you are seeing on the juice label is the naturally-occurring fructose.

Please email if you have any further questions.

In this week's assignment, please see the meal section of the website to examine the protein in your diet. Keep up the great work!

Let's Begin

Protein is made up of amino acids, some of which are essential and some non-essential. When discussing nutrition, essential means that your body can't make it or can't make it in sufficient quantities. If a food contains all the essential amino acids, it is considered a complete protein source. A food that contains only some of the essential amino acids is called an incomplete protein source. As a general rule, plant sources (except soy) are incomplete proteins, and meat (all types), poultry, and fish are complete proteins.

Individuals who consume a vegetarian diet must be careful to pair foods in order to create complete proteins. For example, wheat contains certain amino acids and nuts contain other amino acids: Putting peanut butter on wheat bread makes a complete protein.

Your high school biology class covered protein synthesis or DNA synthesis. You probably remember the DNA helix that looks like a ladder split down the middle. In DNA or protein synthesis, the building blocks are assembled from the proteins you eat. If you don't consume adequate protein, your body can't complete the necessary DNA synthesis. Your hair is the first place low protein intake reveals itself—hair cells have rapid turnover, and without enough protein in the diet, you begin to notice increased hair loss and/or thinning hair. Your diet's protein quality is also vital to a healthy immune system and strong muscles.

Conversely, it is also possible to consume too much protein. One major problem associated with overconsumption of protein is the loss of calcium. And with four calories per gram of protein, it's easy to consume extra calories. Individuals working hard to lose weight without seeing results are often overconsuming protein that the body converts to stored fats.

So, how much protein do you need? Let's look at what we have already learned.

Protein should represent 12–20% of total calories. Using 1,800 calories as an example, we multiply 1,800 by 0.12 and 0.20.

1,800 x 0.12 = 216/4 calories per gram = 54 g.

1,800 x 0.20 = 360/4 calories per gram = 90 g.

There are four calories per gram of protein. Consuming too much or too little can have negative effects on your health.

	Carbohydrates	Protein	Fats
Grain	15g	3g	0–1g
Fruit	15 g	0 g	0 g
Vegetable	5 g	2 g	0 g
Dairy	12 g	8 g	0–8 g
Meat	0 g	7 g	0–8 g
Fat	0 g	0 g	5 g

Protein has a recommended dietary allowance (RDA) establishing the level healthy adults should stay above. The RDA does not ensure adequacy, hence the use of 12–20% of total calories when calculating protein needs.

Go back to Module 7 to look at your calorie needs and then calculate your daily protein needs.

MODULE 8

PROTEINS AND YOU

Review

Balancing a diet is about balancing the nutrients you need <u>that are</u> <u>unique to you</u>. There are as many right answers to a balanced diet as there are people. At the beginning of the book, you started examining your diet with the MyPlate as the working tool to help organize your nutrients. Now you are beginning to look at each nutrient group that makes up the food groups. Last week you looked closer at the total carbohydrates in your diet and determined how much you need and how much you are consuming. This week you will look closer at the protein in your diet.

Let's Begin

Think back to your biology classes and learning about protein synthesis or DNA synthesis. You may have been required to build a helix that looked like someone took a ladder and split it in the middle. In DNA or protein synthesis, the building blocks are provided by the proteins you eat. If you don't consume adequate protein, your body can't complete all the necessary DNA synthesis. Sustained lack of protein is seen first in the hair: Hair cells turn over rapidly, and without enough dietary protein, you'll notice increased hair shedding and overall hair thinning. The protein quality of your diet is also vital to a healthy immune system and strong muscles.

But it is also possible to consume too much protein. One major problem associated with consuming too much protein is calcium loss. Also, with four calories per gram, you can be accidentally consuming extra calories. Too often I have worked with individuals working hard at the gym but not getting the expected results. In some cases the problem was overconsumption of protein converted to fat storage in the body.

So, how much protein do you need? Let's look at what we've already learned.

Protein should comprise between 12–20% of calories, and is calculated the same way. Using 1800 calories as an example, multiply 1800 by 0.12 and 0.20:

$$1800 \times 0.12 = 216/4 \text{ calories per gram} = 54 \text{ gms.}$$

$$1800 \times 0.20 = 360/4 \text{ calories per gram} = 90 \text{ gms.}$$

*Like the carbohydrate, **there are 4 calories per gram of protein.** Consuming too much or too little protein can have negative health effects.*

	Carbohydrate	Protein	Fat
Grain	15gms	3gms	0–1gms
Fruit	15gms	0gms	0gms
Vegetable	5gms	2gms	0gms
Dairy	12gms	8gms	0–8gms
Meat	0gms	7gms	0–8gms
Fat	0gms	0gms	5gms

While there is a recommended dietary allowance (RDA) for protein, it does not insure adequacy, so 12%–20% of total calories is used when calculating protein needs..

MODULE 9

REVIEW

YOU'VE LOOKED AT THE TOTAL CARBOHYDRATES AND protein you consume and realized it can be tough to balance your diet.

The last energy nutrient is fat. We will also be exploring alcohol, which provides calories but is not considered a nutrient.

Let's Begin

A healthy diet should include 25–35% of its total daily calories from fats—this is up from the previously recommended amount of 30%. The majority of fat should come from monounsaturated fat, found in olive oil, canola oil, peanut oil, almonds, avocados, and walnuts. Saturated fat, primarily from animals, should be minimized. The third type is polyunsaturated fat, found primarily in vegetables. So far, except for trans fats, polyunsaturated fat has maintained a healthy position in your diet. Please note, however, that all fats are comprised of the three types of fats—it's just that some are predominantly more one type than another.

Saturated fats should make up no more that 10% of your total daily calories. To determine this, multiply your total daily by 0.10. For example, if you're losing weight and consuming approximately 1,800 calories, then 1,800 x 0.10 = 180 calories.

Because all the information on the food label is in grams (g) or milligrams (mg), you must divide by 9 because there are 9 calories per gram of fat, regardless of fat type. Therefore, total saturated fats each day = 20 grams. Try determining the amount of saturated fat you should consume. If you have high cholesterol or a family history of heart disease, you should limit your saturated fat to 7% of total daily calories. Too much fat in the diet can lead to weight gain, certain forms of cancer and heart disease.

Monounsaturated fat is considered heart-healthy but must still be consumed in a balanced amount. We're frequently encouraged to consume monounsaturated fats for heart health, but there is a limit. Monounsaturated fats like olive or canola oils contain saturated fats and contribute to the daily amount of saturated fat you should be consuming.

Historically, if you had high cholesterol and a family history of heart disease, you were encouraged to avoid eggs, butter, cheese, whole milk, and red meat. To help people stay healthy, the food industry created margarine—a liquid turned into a solid through the process of hydrogenation. This was wonderful because instead of butter from an animal source, a "butter-type" product made from vegetables became an option. Unfortunately, the process of converting a liquid to a solid creates trans fats, which scientists now understand increases the risk for other forms of heart disease and certain forms of cancer.

Manufacturers are now required to list the amount of trans fats on food labels—and your goal amount should be zero.

Some of the functions of fat include:

- Body insulation
- Cushioning organs
- Dissolving fat-soluble vitamins
- Cell structure
- Shiny hair
- Healthy skin
- Facilitating reactions

Fat is also important to the taste and smell of food. If you've ever tried to sauté onions and peppers in water versus olive oil or butter, you will quickly understand: Fat is aromatic and enhances enjoyment of food. It's also the slowest burning of the three energy nutrients and provides a feeling of satiety or fullness.

So, fat is important to your health, and the goal is to consume it in a balanced format where your taste is satisfied and your health is maximized.

MODULE 10

VITAMINS AND MINERALS

Review

You've examined carbohydrates, proteins, and fats and determined the level of each in your diet. These three nutrient groups are known as the energy nutrients or "the macros" because they provide us with calories. Trying to keep the three balanced can feel like a juggling act. Using MyPlate can make the job of balancing your diet much easier.

Let's Begin

Vitamins and minerals are considered non-energy nutrients because they do not provide calories. They are, however, essential, which means you must eat them because your body can't make them or make them in sufficient quantities. Vitamins and minerals can be neither created nor destroyed by living organisms.

Vitamins

Vitamins were originally thought to be "vital amines," or a part of the proteins in our diets. As time passed and research grew, it became apparent that these organic (which means carbon-containing) substances were not proteins. The words were condensed and the "vitamin" group emerged. Nutrition science is young and still evolving: Within the vitamin group, Vitamin D is currently being re-categorized and is now also believed to be a hormone.

Vitamins fall into in water-soluble and fat-soluble categories. Water-soluble vitamins include Vitamin C and all the B vitamins. Fat-soluble vitamins include Vitamins A, D, E, and K. Vitamin D is still included on the list.

Each vitamin plays an important role in your health. For example, the B vitamin folate (also called folacin) is crucial in DNA synthesis: Women trying to conceive are encouraged to ensure the adequate intake of folic acid to prevent neural tube defects such as spina bifida. In 1998, the United States began fortifying foods with folate, which resulted in a significant reduction of babies born with neural tube defects.

Minerals

Your body contains 40 or more minerals, but so far only 15 appear to be dietary essentials. The other necessary minerals are obtained by breathing or via other nutrients in the diet such as protein and vitamins. Like vitamins, minerals are organic substances. The electrical charge minerals carry allows them to bond to other minerals with opposite charges, which explains why minerals are so hard. For example, bones are strong for the same reason that rocks are hard. It is this charge that enables minerals to function as they do.

The electrical current generated by charged minerals can be recorded by an electrocardiogram (EKG). For example, abnormalities in an EKG pattern show potential or past problems in the heart muscle. Because of their charge, minerals can also combine with other substances in food and form highly stable compounds not easily absorbed.

Absorption of zinc from food, for example, can vary from 0–100%, depending on what's attached to it. Zinc can bond with a substance in grains called pyate, making it very difficult for the body to absorb. Zinc in meats, however, is readily absorbed because it is bound to protein.

Calcium, iron, sodium, and potassium are some of the most common dietary minerals. Like vitamins, each mineral is vital for your health.

Let's look at MyPlate and see some of the vitamins and minerals in each group.

- **The starch group provides** many of the necessary B vitamins, including thiamin (B-1), riboflavin (B-2), niacin (B-3), and folate, and the minerals potassium and phosphorus.

- **The fruit group offers** potassium, vitamin B-6, folate, vitamin C, and vitamin A.

- **The vegetable group provides** vitamin A, vitamin K, riboflavin, vitamin B-6, vitamin C, potassium, calcium, and magnesium.

- **The dairy group offers** potassium, phosphorus, calcium, riboflavin, vitamin A, and vitamin D.

- **The meat/protein group provides** thiamine, niacin, vitamin B-6, vitamin B-12, and sulfur.

- **The fat group offers** vitamin A, vitamin D, and vitamin E. (A note about the fat-soluble vitamin K: Although you obtain some vitamin K from green leafy vegetables, much of it is made by microorganisms in our intestines.)

For additional reading on vitamins and minerals, see myplate.gov and www.cdc.gov.

WATER, WATER EVERYWHERE

Review

You've learned about carbohydrates, proteins, fats, vitamins, and minerals and determined the best level of each in your diet. MyPlate helped you balance these nutrients to achieve good health. The last nutrient to examine is the most important: water.

Let's Begin

Depending on the amount of stored fat in your body, you could probably live for about eight weeks without any food. The same is not true for water: Most people can only survive for a few days without water. The human body uses approximately two quarts of water each day just to carry out basic functions, and the body doesn't have any way to store extra water.

When you get on a scale, the majority of your weight is water— anywhere from 50–70%. Muscle contains about 73% water and fat contains about 20%. This explains why people say that when you start exercising and watching your food intake, you lose inches before you lose pounds...muscle weighs more than fat.

Water is responsible for many daily bodily tasks. Most chemical reactions in the body are carried out through water. There is water inside and outside each cell. Water helps regulate body temperature and remove waste products. It is also the basis of saliva and the amniotic fluid that surrounds a fetus.

Water keeps the joints mobile and appears to help start the healing process. Think about the last time you had a blister—what was the first thing you saw? Water.

Estimated daily output of water from your body includes:

Perspiration	2 cups
Respiration	1.7 cups
Urine	5.5 cups
Feces	0.6 cups
Total	10 cups

The minimum recommended daily intake of fluid includes:

Women	11 eight-ounce cups
Men	15 eight-ounce cups

Please note that the recommendation for intake is listed as "fluids"—all fluids, including coffee, tea, soda, and milk are now considered acceptable water replacements. Caffeine found in coffee and tea was previously considered a diuretic and those drinks were not thought to be water replacements, but that did not hold up in research. While caffeine *is* a diuretic, its effect is not strong enough to discount the caffeinated beverage's water content.

Additional water needed daily comes from food. Water is found in abundance in fruits and vegetables. Those with the highest water content include romaine lettuce, tomatoes, zucchini, asparagus, cantaloupe, grapefruit, honeydew melon, and orange juice. Other foods rich in water include cottage cheese, tofu, water-packed tuna, potatoes, corn, rice, hard-cooked eggs, bananas, beans, skinless chicken, pasta, ice cream, baked salmon, and cod.

Water deficiency is called dehydration. If you become dehydrated, you'll notice that urine output becomes increasingly darker in color and develops a strong odor. As time passes, the kidneys produce less and less urine in an attempt to regulate the body's water balance. Other dehydration signs include stronger thirst, loss of appetite, lagging pace, impatience, weariness, nausea, headache, and tingling in arms, hands and feet.

Thirst is the message your body sends when more fluids are required. It's important to note that your body is approximately 1% dehydrated when it sends the thirst signal. Sports research has demonstrated that by the time an athlete is 2% dehydrated, his/her performance is down 10%. This is true for everyone, so it's best to drink all day and not get to the point of thirst. A pre- and post-workout weigh-in is recommended for athletes or others exercising. You should then drink water or sports drinks until the lost weight is restored.

It is possible to get *too much* fluid as well. This is called water toxicity or water intoxication. This occurs most often when water intake is not accompanied by sufficient electrolytes.

Very few people are at risk of water intoxication as this requires consuming many quarts of water each day.

A final hydration point: In addition to eating adequate food during the day for maximum energy, it's equally important to have adequate fluid. If you don't usually drink much during the day, try to drink four to six eight-ounce glasses of fluid by 4 PM and see if your energy improves.

MODULE 12

NUTRITION FOR PHYSICAL FITNESS

Review

We've examined carbohydrates, proteins, fats, vitamins, minerals, and water and determined the optimal level of each in your personal diet. Continue to use MyPlate to help you balance these nutrients and achieve good health. You're now positioned to explore how to change your basic pattern to achieve optimal success in your workouts.

Let's Begin

Please remember that you will achieve the maximum benefit of any activity or sports nutrition intervention only if you have a balanced diet to begin with—otherwise, it's like putting a new Band-Aid on a dirty wound. So, with that said, please be sure you consume all your food groups daily and drink adequate fluids.

Nutrition for physical fitness involves fueling for activities, both aerobic and anaerobic (the body's energy-producing pathways).

In the physical fitness world, aerobic or cardio exercise refers raising your heart rate into an age-related target zone. The word aerobic itself means "with oxygen." The aerobic movement was started by Dr. Kenneth Cooper in the 1950s when he began his research on military men. His research established the age-related target heart-rate zones we use today. When he began, Dr. Cooper recommended elevating the heart rate into the target zone and staying there for 20 minutes three times a week. At that time, the average person walked about 18,000 steps daily; the average person now walks only 4,000–6,000 steps daily, and with a minimum recommendation of 10,000 steps. This provides some insight into why the daily recommendation for physical activity continues to increase. Adults should be physically active for 30–90 minutes on most days, depending on personal goals.

Anaerobic exercise, or strength training, involves toning or building muscle. Anaerobic means "without oxygen." You break your muscles down each time you work them; muscle is toned and built as it heals and recovers. A personal trainer or, if needed, a physical therapist can assist you in achieving personal goals and preventing injuries.

As we already know, a basic diet consists of 58% carbohydrates, 30% fats, and 12% protein. If you play a sport or work out regularly, it's necessary to change these percentages to 60/20/20 due to the increased need for fuel and repair materials. Carbohydrates are the fuel needed to step up activity, and they function just like adding more gas to your car when taking a long road trip. Proteins are the repair materials for the muscle cells.

Your body stores carbohydrates in a form called glycogen, the primary fuel for muscles during exercise. Eventually, the more time you spend in aerobic exercise, the more fat is used for energy—but always in the presence of glycogen. Research shows there's a two-hour window after aerobic exercise ends in which you can eat carbohydrates and replace glycogen in order to provide good muscle energy the next day.

Here's the quick and simple calculation for glycogen replacement from Barbara Day's book <u>High Performance Demands a High Performance Diet</u>. You will want to be between 50%–75%

Your weight in pounds:	_____	lbs.
Multiply your weight x 0.50	=	grams for recovery
Multiply your weight x 0.75	=	grams for recovery

Some foods/beverages suggested for that two-hour post-exercise window include juices, sports drinks, baked potatoes, pasta, rice, and milkshakes. Remember that the carbohydrates in these replacement foods count toward your daily total carbohydrate intake.

After an anaerobic workout, you must replace proteins to provide the building blocks for muscle repair. Like carbohydrates, proteins also have a window of time for optimal replacement, 30–60 minutes after the muscle resistance exercise ends. To discover your protein need, calculate the difference between your 12% and 20% need. For example, if you weigh 150 pounds and are maintaining your weight (15 cals/pound) then 12% = 68 grams and 20% = 113 grams. The difference is 44 grams. Some foods such as Greek yogurt provide complete proteins and include dairy and protein. One cup of fat-free Greek yogurt contains approximately 120 calories, 9 grams of carbohydrates and 20 grams of protein—a great and easy start to the 44 gram replacement.

For fluids, it's generally suggested that if your workout is an hour or less, water is your best bet. Throughout the 1980s and 90s, research suggested that sports drinks should replace water after about 15 minutes. However, long story short, the research came from the Gatorade Institute—a clear bias. A simple estimate for post-workout fluid replacement is to weigh in pre- and post-workout and then drink until your weight is restored.

Here are some general guidelines for maintaining hydration during physical exercise, also from Barbara Day:

- Drink 16 ounces of fluid two hours before the event.

- Drink 8 ounces of fluid 15–30 minutes before the event.

- Drink 6 ounces of fluid every 15–20 minutes during the event if possible.

- Choose a cool drink (40–50 degrees).

- Remember that one gulp or mouthful is about an ounce of fluid.

MODULE 13

ANTIOXIDANTS: ARE THEY REALLY IMPORTANT TO YOUR HEALTH?

ANTIOXIDANTS ARE TYPICALLY COMPOUNDS THAT CAN donate electrons to oxidized compounds, making them more stable.

Adequate consumption of antioxidants protects your cells against the formation of free radicals. These free radicals have been linked with cardiovascular disease, cancer, skin aging, and arthritis.

Antioxidants are important to health and prevent and manage disease processes in the body. While there are upwards of 600 different compounds under study for their antioxidant properties, some of the better-known and studied antioxidants include lycopene, lutein, and the carotenes, all part of the carotenoid family.

The focus of this module will be to explore these pigmentations, which will hopefully give you more reasons to eat your fruits and vegetables daily. Remember, the roots of tomorrow's diseases are put down today. Let's pull those roots before they take hold!

Lycopene

Lycopene is the bright red color found in tomatoes and other red fruit and is found in the diet mainly in foods prepared with tomato sauce. Lycopene is also instrumental in the development of other colors in our plant foods. Due to its strong color, it is frequently used as a food coloring. Lycopene is not considered an essential nutrient for humans at this time.

Absorbed through food, lycopene is transported to the liver, adrenal glands, and testes. Fruits and vegetables high in lycopene include tomatoes, watermelon, pink grapefruit, pink guava, papaya, red bell pepper, wolfberry (goji), and rosehip. Ironically, because of the way lycopene is carried, its richest sources are found in processed tomato products such as pasteurized tomato juice, soup, sauce, and ketchup.

Lycopene is fat-soluble, which means it's absorbed with fat. Using fats and oils in your meal will enhance the absorption of any present lycopene.

Lutein

Lutein is orange-red and was traditionally used in chicken feed to create the familiar yellow color of broiler chicken skin. Lutein is found in leafy green vegetables such as spinach and kale. Turnip greens, collard greens, romaine lettuce, broccoli, zucchini, corn, garden peas, and Brussels sprouts are also good sources. Lutein is also found in egg yolks and animal fats. While no recommended dietary allowance exists for lutein, positive effects have been seen at intake levels of 6 mg/day.

Lutein has been shown to play a role in protecting the eyes from oxidative stress and high-energy light and decrease the risk of age-related macular degeneration.

Carotene

Carotene is actually several related plant-based substances. Animals cannot produce carotene—it must be consumed. Carotene is responsible for the orange color in foods and for the orange color in dry fall foliage. Beta-carotene is one of the best-known carotenoids. Carotene is digested, absorbed, stored in the liver and body fat, and converted to Vitamin A if necessary. Vitamin A is necessary for vision. Beta-carotene is currently being studied for its role in cognition, photosensitivity, and nanotechnology.

Carotene-rich foods include sweet potatoes, carrots, goji berries, cantaloupe, mango, apricots, spinach, kale, collard greens, broccoli, parsley, winter squash, and pumpkin.

Continue to balance your diet and include fruits and vegetables daily.

NAVIGATING THE GROCERY STORE

Review

We've examined carbohydrates, proteins, fats, vitamins, minerals, water, and antioxidants and determined the optimal level of each in your personal diet. Grocery shopping for food to provide these nutrients can be challenging. So how best to approach it?

Let's Begin

Grocery stores exist to sell food and beverages *and* to make money. Keep in mind that a grocery store is designed to encourage impulse buying. Rule one is never grocery shop hungry—you *will* buy things you don't need or want if your stomach is empty.

Endcaps (the shelves at the end of each aisle) are set up for impulse buying. Plus, the most popular and high-sodium/high-sugar foods are placed at eye level. You frequently have to work harder—bend down, get on tiptoe up—to see healthier, balanced choices. Almost all of the whole and unprocessed foods are located on the perimeter of the store. If you're striving to prepare more nutritious foods, shop more on the perimeter, and remember that these foods take longer to prepare and cook.

Most grocery stores take you through the produce section first. Choose as many different colors as possible. When you exit the produce section, your cart should have the makings of an artist's palette. Look for freshness and richness of color in your products.

Is organic worth the higher cost? If you're focused on nutrition, no. Research shows there's no significant nutritional difference between organic and non-organic produce. But if you are trying to minimize your consumption of pesticides and other chemicals, then the answer is yes.

As you make your way to the back of the store you will find the meat section, including beef, poultry, pork, and fish. Try to choose the leanest cuts possible, identifiable by the least visible fat. The more marbling, the higher the calories and saturated fat. Remember to have fish three times weekly if possible.

As you shop, remember that there are no good or bad foods, only balanced or unbalanced diets.

Moving into dairy, again, choose lower-fat products as tolerated. When looking at yogurt, try to identify those yogurts that contain live active cultures. Active cultures, or probiotics, are the good bacteria in the yogurt. (Just an FYI: Probiotics live on the prebiotics in consumed fiber. If you're eating a probiotic-rich but low-fiber diet, you're defeating the purpose of consuming probiotics.)

When looking at breads and cereals, choose those that contain whole grains. It doesn't help to eat 12-grain bread if all the grains are refined. Fiber intake should come in at 20–35 grams/day. When choosing bread, pick one with 2 g or more of fiber per slice; when choosing cereal, pick 5 g or more of fiber per serving.

When moving to the interior of the store, be aware of the sodium content of foods. Interior aisles contain more processed, higher-additive, higher-sodium, less nutritious foods. Recommended sodium intake per day is 2,300 mg. It's very easy to consume excess sodium when eating on the run and having many prepared quick foods.

Continue improving the balance of your diet!

MEET THE AUTHORS

Richard R. Terry, DO, MBA

Dr. Richard Terry is a highly-accomplished family physician and esteemed Professor of Family Medicine at the Lake Erie College of Osteopathic Medicine (LECOM). He holds board certification in family medicine and is the founding Dean of LECOM at Elmira, the first and sole medical school in the Southern Tier of New York. Presently, Dr. Terry assumes the vital roles of Associate Dean of Academic Affairs at LECOM at Elmira and Chief Academic Officer of the LECOM Consortium for Academic Excellence (LCAE).

With an impressive tenure spanning more than two decades, Dr. Terry possesses extensive expertise in medical education. He frequently delivers lectures on a wide range of educational and health-related topics, both at regional and national levels. His exceptional teaching abilities have garnered national recognition, and his exemplary practice in treating weight management conditions extends over 25 years. As an osteopathic physician, Dr. Terry strongly advocates for holistic approaches and lifestyle management strategies to enhance the overall well-being of patients. Moreover, he is deeply committed to educating the next generation of osteopathic physicians, imparting invaluable knowledge and skills to shape their future practices.

www.tomorrowsweigh.com

Helen E. Battisti, PhD, RDN

Dr. Battisti is a Registered Dietitian Nutritionist (RDN) and a health promotion specialist. She maintains a consulting business working with athletes, individuals and organizations looking to improve their performance, health and productivity through enhanced nutrition.

For over 30 years, Helen was a full-time Assistant Professor at Marywood University in the department of Nutrition and Dietetics, Athletic Training and Exercise Science, Scranton, Pennsylvania, as well as a clinical RDN with Endwell Family Physicians, Endwell, New York. She was the lead RDN at a research site that investigated the Wegovy medication for the treatment of obesity. She has numerous publications reflecting her ongoing commitment to helping better understand obesity, the causes, and solutions. She continues to share her knowledge through presentations and training.

Dr. Battisti holds a certificate in pediatric and adult weight management from the Academy of Nutrition and Dietetics. In addition to working in the area of health and weight management, she has personally experienced the challenges having been obese as a teenager and maintaining her weight throughout her adult life.

www.tomorrowsweigh.com | www.spnod.com

Francis L. Battisti, PhD, MSW

Dr. Battisti is a nationally-recognized speaker on topics of health enhancement, conflict resolution, resilience, and Appreciative Inquiry. As a psychotherapist, his keen appreciation for the uniqueness of individuals allows him to share the client's journey. He has presented to audiences throughout the United States, Mexico, and Colombia. His research focuses on families and new methodologies for health enhancement. His unique area of inquiry includes the relationship of children and their fathers.

At SUNY Broome Community College in Binghamton, NY, he is an emeritus psychology professor and past Executive Vice President and Chief Academic Officer. He is a Distinguished Professor with the State University of New York and has been admitted to the Distinguished Professor Academy. He is the author of Checchino: A Father and Son Journey Toward Dusk.

www.tomorrowsweigh.com | www.battistimanagement.com

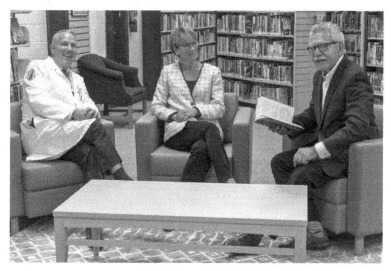

Left to right: Drs. R. Terry, H. Battisti, F. Battisti